D1474917

EVALUATING COMMUNITY COLLABORATIONS

Thomas E. Backer is president of the Human Interaction Research Institute, a Los Angeles-based nonprofit center for research and intervention on innovation and change. He is also associate clinical professor of medical psychology at the UCLA School of Medicine. A psychologist, his life work is devoted to helping people, organizations, and communities meet the challenges of innovation and change. He has three central interests: the human dynamics of change for both individuals and organizations; use of strategic planning and other problem-solving methods to meet the challenges of change; and the psychology of creativity. He conducts research, writes, teaches, and consults in all three areas—concentrating on work that improves services for vulnerable populations, and on enhancing nonprofit arts and culture programs.

He is the author of more than 400 books, articles, and research reports. *Dissemination and Utilization Strategies for Foundations: Adding Value to Grantmaking*, and *Reviewing the Behavioral Science Knowledge Base on Technology Transfer* (coedited with Susan L. David and Gerald Soucy of the National Institute on Drug Abuse) are his most recent books. He is also the author of three recently completed research studies of innovations in philanthropy, all commissioned by the John S. and James L. Knight Foundation.

Dr. Backer won the 1989 Mrs. Swanson Award of the Knowledge Utilization Society, for his longtime research and consultation on labor and management responses to the AIDS health crisis. He was also awarded the 1987 Consulting Psychology Research Award of the Division of Consulting Psychology, American Psychological Association, and its 2001 RHR International Award for Excellence in Consultation.

EVALUATING
COMMUNITY
COLLABORATIONS

Thomas E. Backer, PhD
Editor

 Springer Publishing Company

Springer Publishing Company, Inc.
536 Broadway
New York, NY 10012-3955

Acquisitions Editor: Sheri W. Sussman
Production Editor: Jeanne W. Libby
Cover design by Joanne E. Honigman

03 04 05 06 07/5 4 3 2 1

Library of Congress Cataloging-in-Publication Data

Evaluating Community Collaborations / Thomas E. Backer, editor.
    p. cm.
  Includes bibliographical references and index.
  ISBN 0-8261-2185-3
    1. Human services--United States--Citizen participation--Evaluation. 2. Community organization--United States--Citizen participation--Evaluation. 3. Community health services--United States--Citizen participation--Evaluation. 4. Evaluation research (Social action programs) 5. Cooperation--United States. I. Backer, Thomas E.

  HV91.E786 2003
  361.2'5--dc22

                                         2003057357

Printed in the United States of America by Integrated Book Technology.

This volume was prepared by the Human Interaction Research Institute with support from the Substance Abuse and Mental Health Services Administration (SAMHSA), U.S. Department of Health and Human Services (HHS) under Contract No. 00M00851401D. The content of the volume does not necessarily reflect the views or policies of SAMHSA or HHS.

Contents

Contributors

John Bare is director of program development and evaluation for the John S. and James L. Knight Foundation. He is responsible for designing, managing, and reporting on a variety of research and planning efforts. He has led the way on using evaluation and planning resources to improve Knight Foundation's effectiveness. Dr. Bare's contributions include innovative "what works" toolkits now in use in several Knight communities, and an analytic framework to describe risk levels in grant making. In 1998, he launched the Community Indicators project, to create and track quality-of-life indicators in the 26 communities the Foundation seeks to affect through its local grant making.

Before joining the Knight Foundation in 1997, Dr. Bare worked as a research consultant for news organizations such as *U.S. News & World Report*, the *Omaha World-Herald*, and Cleveland's *Plain Dealer*. He worked as a writer and researcher for the Education Statistics Services Institute in Washington, DC, and as a columnist for 8 years for *The Chapel Hill* (North Carolina) *Herald*. In 1995, Dr. Bare received his PhD in mass communication research from the University of North Carolina at Chapel Hill, where he was a Freedom Forum journalism scholar and a fellow with the Washington Center for Politics and Journalism.

Stephen B. Fawcett is director of the Kansas University Work Group, Kansas Health Foundation, and University Distinguished Professor, Department of Human Development. Professor Fawcett uses behavioral science and community development methods to help understand and improve health and social concerns of importance to communities.

A former VISTA volunteer, Dr. Fawcett worked as a community organizer in public housing and low-income neighborhoods. He has been honored as a fellow in both Division 27 (community psychology) and Division 25 (experimental analysis of behavior) of the American Psychological Association. He received the Distinguished Practice Award of the Society for Community Research and Action and the Higuchi/Endowment Award for Applied Sciences. He is coauthor of more than 100 articles and book chapters and several books in the areas of community/public health, child/youth health and development, and community development.

Dr. Fawcett has been a scholar-in-residence at the Institute of Medicine of the National Academy of Sciences and is a member of the Board on Health Promotion and Disease Prevention. He has consulted with a number of private foundations and national organizations, including the John D. and Catherine T. MacArthur Foundation, the Ewing Marion Kauffman Foundation, the California Wellness Foundation, the U.S. Commission on National and Community Service, and the U.S. Centers for Disease Control and Prevention.

Vincent T. Francisco is associate director of the Work Group on Health Promotion and Community Development; assistant research professor with the Schieffelbusch Institute for Life Span Studies; courtesy assistant professor with the Department of Human Development and Family Life, University of Kansas; and adjunct assistant professor with the Department of Preventive Medicine, University of Kansas Medical School. Dr. Francisco is primarily interested in research in community development, especially as it enhances community integration and support and work toward empowerment of marginalized groups. He is interested in the provision of technical support for the development of coalitions and evaluation of community-based intervention programs focusing on adolescent development, reduction of risk for teen substance abuse, assaultive violence, teen parenthood, and chronic/cardiovascular diseases.

In his current position, Dr. Francisco works with ethnic minority communities and the general population, to prevent a variety of problems in living. Dr. Francisco has experience providing technical assistance and support for universal and targeted initiatives in communities, including native Hawaiian and Asian American communities, Native American reservations such as the Jicarilla Apache Tribe, African American communities such as mid-south Chicago (Bronzeville), as well as immigrant communities in the northeastern and midwestern United States.

Prior to his current position at the University of Kansas, Dr. Francisco did research in behavioral medicine at the Brown University School of Medicine. In addition, Dr. Francisco also worked at a residential treatment facility for youth in central New Hampshire. As assistant director of this facility, Dr. Francisco had primary responsibility for the intake, admission, and discharge of clients in all programs, as well as administrative functioning and licensing of the facility.

Nancy G. Guerra is professor of psychology at the University of California at Riverside and Associate Director of the Robert Presley Center for Crime and Justice Studies; she also is senior research scientist, Human Interaction Research Institute. She is the principal investigator on the evaluation of a

Safe Schools/Healthy Students grant (to the Riverside Unified School District), funded by the Substance Abuse and Mental Health Services Administration, and is the principal investigator/director of the Southern California Consortium for Youth Violence Prevention, funded by the Centers for Disease Control and Prevention (CDC). She has served on several editorial boards and grant review committees, and is currently a member of the National Institute of Mental Health (NIMH) review group on Prevention and Health Behavior. She was also a member of the President's Coordinating Council on Juvenile Justice from 1994 to 1999.

Dr. Guerra has published numerous professional articles in journals and chapters in books. Most of her work has focused on youth violence prevention and has addressed issues in collaboration, programming, and evaluation. With funding from NIMH and CDC, she has developed and evaluated several large-scale youth violence prevention programs, including the Yes I Can program, Metropolitan Area Child Study, and Viewpoints intervention. For the past 5 years, she has provided technical assistance to 19 youth violence prevention planning and implementation projects funded by the John S. and James L. Knight Initiative to Promote Youth Development and Prevent Youth Violence. She has also recently completed a review of the violence prevention portfolio of the Interamerican Development Bank, which provides large loans to countries in Latin America and the Caribbean for community-based violence prevention programs.

Cynthia D. Kunz is senior research scientist, Human Interaction Research Institute, based in Arlington, Virginia, and an institutional mediator in private practice. She also is president of Kunz and Company. She specializes in institutional conflict prevention, resolution and process improvements in workplace and labor cases, cases arising in not-for-profit and service-providing organizations, and in federal policy, grantee, and contractor matters. A substantial part of Ms. Kunz's mediation practice has involved four, often interrelated, subject matter areas: substance abuse policy, workplace employment and labor management cooperation, health care and disability issues, and business process improvements.

Ms. Kunz served in several staff advisory roles to both regional and national programs of the National Institute on Drug Abuse, which addressed the knowledge and skill development of substance abuse program administrators and counselors and their integration within the allied health fields, including the Central, Southwest, and Western Regional Support Centers and the National Career Development Center. She served as part of the staff team for the Department of Labor's Management Assistance and Training system, developing courses and training administrators and staff from the 102 Job Corps Centers in substance abuse prevention programming and crisis intervention.

For the Human Interaction Research Institute, Ms. Kunz has served as co-project director on several projects, including two current projects for the National 4-H Council. She also collaborates with the Institute in its role as one of the six key partners operating the National Center for the Advancement of Prevention, funded by the Center for Substance Abuse Prevention.

Alex J. Norman is senior research scientist, Human Interaction Research Institute, and professor emeritus of social welfare at UCLA's School of Public Policy and Social Research, where he was chair of the Planning and Administration Department. He holds a bachelor's degree in sociology and business administration from Morris Brown College in Atlanta, Georgia (his home town) and a master's degree in social work from Atlanta University, both historically Black colleges and universities. He holds a doctorate in social welfare from UCLA, as its first graduate in that field, and was on the faculty for 16 years.

Prior to joining the UCLA faculty, Dr. Norman was director of the Departments of Urban Affairs and Social Welfare at University Extension, and, prior to that position, was a social work practitioner for 10 years in Philadelphia, Atlanta, and Los Angeles. He has also served in an executive capacity in a number of community development and youth-serving organizations.

He has conducted research in the United States, Canada, England, Wales, and Scotland, on self-help among African descendents, and conducted comparative studies on community development in the United States and the United Kingdom. He has published journal articles and review chapters in both the United States and the UK on various topics in social planning, organization and management development, interethnic conflict, and mutual aid.

Currently, Dr. Norman serves as an independent consultant to private and public organizations in strategic planning, organization development, conflict management, community development, and managing multicultural environments.

Jerry A. Schultz is associate director of the Kansas University Work Group and adjunct assistant professor, Department of Preventive Medicine. Dr. Schultz holds a PhD in anthropology and an MA in medical anthropology from the University of Kansas. He works primarily with issues involving building capacity of urban neighborhoods to solve local problems, understanding systems change, and evaluating community health and development initiatives.

Dr. Schultz has spent several years as part of the team that is building the Community Tool Box (CTB), an on-line resource for community building. His primary responsibility has been content development for the CTB. Dr. Schultz has coauthored numerous articles on evaluation, empowerment, and community development. He has been a consultant to several foundations, community coalitions, and state agencies.

In addition to his work in community health and development, Dr. Schultz has studied East Asian and Native American culture and history, producing several documentaries on these subjects. Dr. Schultz is a fellow of the Society for Applied Anthropology.

Abraham Wandersman is a professor of psychology at the University of South Carolina—Columbia. He received his PhD from Cornell University in the following areas of specialization: social psychology, environmental psychology, and social organization and change. He was interim codirector of the Institute for Families in Society at the University of South Carolina.

Dr. Wandersman has performed research on environmental issues and community responses. He also performs research and program evaluation on citizen participation in community organizations and coalitions and on interagency collaboration. He is a coauthor of *Prevention Plus III* and a coeditor of *Empowerment Evaluation: Knowledge and Tools for Self Assessment and Accountability* and of many other books and articles. In 1998, he received the Myrdal Award for Evaluation Practice from the American Evaluation Association. In 2000, he was elected president of Division 27 of the American Psychological Association (community psychology), the Society for Community Research and Action. In 2001, he and his coauthors received a presidential prize for mainstreaming evaluation from the American Evaluation Association for the paper *Pie a la Mode: Mainstreaming Evaluation and Accountability in Each Program of Every County in a Statewide School Readiness Initiative.*

Recently, Dr. Wandersman was engaged in work with the governor's office on a statewide initiative for improving school readiness, involving county partnerships in the 46 counties of South Carolina. The work includes developing and evaluating the results-oriented grant-making and grant implementation system that is being used in the initiative. As part of this initiative, he created a workbook, training, and technical assistance strategy that will help each program achieve its intended outcomes.

Tom Wolff is with Community Partners, Inc., and is a nationally recognized consultant on coalition building and community development, with more than

30 years' experience training and consulting for organizations, foundations, grassroots community groups, and governments in Massachusetts and across North America.

Dr. Wolff's writings on coalition building include the popular workbook, *From the Ground Up*, a workbook on coalition building and community development, as well as *The Spirit of the Coalition* (with Bill Berkowitz), published by the American Public Health Association in 2000. He coauthored *Outreach Works: Strategies for Expanding Health Access in Communities* in 2001. A recent article edited by Dr. Wolff, "Community Coalition Building: Contemporary Practice and Research," was published as a special edition of the *American Journal of Community Psychology* in April 2001. He has also been the editor of *The Community Catalyst* and the *Healthy Communities Massachusetts* newsletters produced by AHEC/Community Partners.

Dr. Wolff is senior consultant for AHEC/Community Partners, a technical assistance and training program for those involved in coalition building and community development. This program has started and consulted with dozens of community coalitions across the state. He has now expanded this work into a unique state network—Healthy Communities Massachusetts—linking innovative community-building efforts in cities and towns.

Dr. Wolff is a fellow of the American Psychological Association, which granted him its 1985 National Career Award for Distinguished Contributions to Practice in community psychology and its 1993 Henry V. McNeil award for innovation in community mental health. He received his undergraduate degree from Clark University and his PhD from the University of Rochester.

Foreword

What's the News About Community Collaborations?
The Good, the Not-So-Good, and a Cautiously Optimistic Forecast

Abe Wandersman

As this volume and other recent publications affirm (e.g., Kreuter, Lezin, & Young, 2000; Roussos & Fawcett, 2000), community collaborations are a popular mechanism for addressing public health (mental and medical health) problems. In many cases, if grantees wish to be funded, collaboration with community partners is required by government and foundation funders.

In this age of accountability, the kinds of questions asked about results of these collaborations, whether voluntary or required for funding, are, for example, Is the collaboration working? and, Does it lead to measurable outcomes and impacts? Funders and grantees are asked, about program implementation and process, for example, Why are collaborations so hard to do? and, What can we do to make collaborations work better?

Related to these accountability questions, there is good news and not-so-good news regarding the results of community collaborations (for a fuller discussion, see Wandersman & Florin, in press). The good news is that there are examples of collaborations that have shown positive results. Research-driven prevention is typically directed by university or research institute professionals who often use experimental or quasi-experimental designs. Research-driven, community-level interventions that have involved collaboration between community partners have shown results in areas such as substance abuse prevention and heart disease prevention (e.g., Pentz et al., 1989; Backer & Rogers, 1993).

Community-driven prevention, on the other hand, is owned and operated by organizations in the community, and is conducted every day in schools and other community settings that reach millions of people. Community interventions that involve collaboration between community partners have shown results in areas such as substance abuse prevention, delinquency, and maternal and child health outcomes (e.g., Galano & Huntington, 1997).

The not-so-good news is that systematic reviews and cross-site evaluations of community collaborations show a modest and mixed record of results. Sometimes they have demonstrated results, and many times they have not (see, for instance, Roussos & Fawcett, 2000; Kreuter et al., 2000). This volume, in fact, presents many of the challenges—technical, political, and resource-driven, among others—that help to account for these inconsistent results.

My cautiously optimistic forecast from all of the preceding (and this volume is part of my forecast) begins with this observation: Traditional evaluation methods aim to use experimental and quasi-experimental designs to objectively and neutrally answer the question, Did the community collaboration achieve results? What funders and communities have generally found is the not-so-good news just described. This is important information, but it has limited utility in helping collaborations achieve results. Empowerment evaluation may be of some value here.

Empowerment evaluation methods and tools are being developed to increase the capacity of community agencies and collaborations to deliver evidence-based programs more effectively to achieve results. Therefore, empowerment evaluation is becoming a popular approach with funders and grantees.

In empowerment evaluation, the purpose of the evaluation is to enhance program quality and the ability to achieve results by increasing the capacity of program stakeholders (any individual, group, or organization that has an interest in how well a program functions) to plan, implement, and evaluate their own programs (Fetterman, 2001; Fetterman, Kaftarian, & Wandersman, 1996; Wandersman, 1999).

Wandersman et al. (2002) have presented the most recent overview of principles of empowerment evaluation. Here are several that are relevant to this volume:

- Empowerment evaluators help program stakeholders (e.g., staff, consumers) develop the capacity to plan, implement, and evaluate their own programs.
- The results of an empowerment evaluation can be evaluated or judged. Outcomes are an important feature of empowerment evaluation and can be objective (e.g., school attendance, dropout rates, incidents of

student violence). An empowerment evaluation can and should be interested in measuring objective outcomes.

- Empowerment evaluation can be used in a complementary fashion with an external evaluation.
- Empowerment evaluation can and should be used for continuous quality improvement.

My colleagues and I have been engaged in a number of empowerment evaluations. We are currently involved with one in South Carolina. The Spartanburg Boys & Girls Club is the lead agency in a collaborative effort to expand proven programs to new sites, so that more club member families have access to these innovative programs.

This combination of best-practice services has created a vertical integration of programs—one targeting parents (Parent University), a program targeting school-age youth (local Boys & Girls Clubs and the TEEN Supreme Center with its enhanced programs), and a program targeting the health and development of preschool youth (Parents as Teachers). Families taking advantage of two or more of these services have increased opportunities to develop the characteristics (e.g., usefulness, competence, belonging, and influence) that will enable them to overcome risk factors and thrive as Spartanburg citizens.

Instead of the Boys & Girls Club offering all of the programs on its own and building them from scratch, it developed a collaborative effort to bring existing agencies that were engaged in best-practice programs to expand their programs into the Boys & Girls Club sites. This involves a great deal of collaboration and some adaptation of the programs. The local funder funded an empowerment evaluation of this initiative. The collaboration was responsible for carrying out most of the process and outcome evaluation. Our roles included helping to set up evaluation plans and a web-based data collection system, commenting on reports written by initiative staff, consulting on the content and best practices of individual programs, and evaluating the strengths and areas of improvement of the collaborative experience of the partners. The staff was responsible for collecting data and writing reports about process and outcomes.

Empowerment evaluation is not a panacea. Since it is a relatively new approach, evidence of its effectiveness, so far, is largely anecdotal and qualitative. Empowerment evaluation has its benefits and costs. It requires that practitioners and other stakeholders develop evaluation. That is why this volume is so helpful.

We know that for any *intervention* to succeed, whether at the individual level (e.g., therapy) or organizational level (e.g., violence prevention programs for a school), it is necessary to have both *good intervention content and a good structure that facilitates its delivery.* For example, achieving therapeutic outcomes requires both the use of evidence-based treatment strategies and treatment delivery from a therapist. Good *prevention* programs catalyzed by any organization, including collaborations, require the same. Federal agencies have promoted the use of evidence-based practices by community agencies and collaborations. Metaphorically, the evidence-based practices are the serum, the magic bullet, that will make people better or vaccinate them from disease.

Good progress has been made in developing empowerment evaluation methods for building the capacity of community stakeholders to better plan, implement, and self-evaluate programs (Fetterman, 2001). Wandersman et al. (2000) developed a system called Getting to Outcomes, which is a results-based accountability approach that uses 10 accountability questions, and how to answer them, to help practitioners achieve results. Empowerment evaluation is one of its roots. This volume contributes important additions in this arena, by providing methods for using data (e.g., the chapter by Francisco, Schultz, & Fawcett) and working with evaluators (Guerra's chapter). In sum, methods and tools for improving the planning, implementing, and evaluation of programs are being developed to help practitioners (this is refining the content or serum).

We need to know what structures support (or undermine) the delivery of the program—the community collaboration. In our metaphor, it is the mechanism that purchases the serum, delivers the serum (hypodermic needle), and injects it in the right place at the right time.

We need a *set of empowerment evaluation methods and tools that help community collaborations become more effective and efficient organizationally.* Collaborations are hard work. By definition, they bring together *diverse* partners with multiple agendas. This volume makes major new contributions that relate to the empowerment evaluation philosophy. It provides concepts (e.g., chapters by Backer and by Backer & Kunz) and methods and tools for collaborations to use to build their capacity to become more effective and efficient organizationally (e.g., chapters by Wolff and by Norman).

I am optimistic because we have the knowledge and tools in this volume. I am cautious because knowledge is not the same as utilization. It is up to you.

REFERENCES

Backer, T. E., & Rogers, E. M. (Eds.). (1993). *Organizational aspects of health communication campaigns: What works?* Newbury Park, CA: Sage.

Fetterman, D., Kaftarian, S., & Wandersman, A. (1996). *Empowerment evaluation: Knowledge and tools for self-assessment and accountability.* Thousand Oaks, CA: Sage.

Fetterman, D. M. (2001). *Foundations of empowerment evaluation.* Thousand Oaks, CA: Sage.

Galano, J., & Huntington, L. (1997). *Healthy families partnership evaluation: A summary.* Hampton, VA: Healthy Families Partnership.

Kreuter, M. W., Lezin, N. A., & Young, L. A. (2000). Evaluating community-based collaborative mechanisms: Implications for practitioners. *Health Promotion Practice, 1*(1), 49–63.

Pentz, M. A., et al. (1989). A multicommunity trial for primary prevention of adolescent drug abuse: Effects on drug use prevalence. *Journal of the American Medical Association, 261*(22), 3259–3266.

Roussos, S. T., & Fawcett, S. B. (2000). A review of collaborative partnerships as a strategy for improving community health. *Annual Review of Public Health, 21,* 369–402.

Wandersman, A. (1999). Framing the evaluation of the health and human service programs in community settings: Assessing progress. *New Directions for Evaluation, 83,* 95–102.

Wandersman, A., & Florin, P. (in press). Community interventions and effective prevention. *American Psychologist.*

Wandersman, A., Imm, P., Chinman, M., & Kaftarian, S. (2000). Getting to outcomes: A results-based approach to accountability. *Evaluation and Program Planning, 23,* 389–395.

Wandersman, A., et al. (2002, June). *Principles of empowerment evaluation.* Paper presented at Chicago Conference on Capturing Theory and Methodology in Participatory Research.

Acknowledgments

This volume was the inspiration of Dr. Malcolm Gordon of the Substance Abuse and Mental Health Services Administration's Center for Mental Health Services (CMHS), and first thanks are due to him for suggesting that the Human Interaction Research Institute create the work as part of our evaluation of the CMHS School and Community Action Grant Program, which funds projects that make prominent use of collaborations in promoting community change, and which seeks to evaluate their impact. We also thank each of our authors, who collectively represent the leadership of both the academic and practice sides of collaboration and its evaluation. At our Institute, I would like to thank Elizabeth Howard and U. Sue Koone, who shepherded the project through its early stages, and Adryan Russ, who capably managed the later editorial work on this volume.

CHAPTER 1

Evaluating Community Collaborations: An Overview

Thomas E. Backer

Collaborations, which bring organizations together in a community to implement or improve an innovative program, or to change a policy or procedure, have become a central strategy for promoting community change. Funders require them; nonprofits see them as useful solutions to their problems of declining resources and increasing complexity (including multicultural issues); and communities demand them as evidence that key stakeholders are coming together to address problems of mutual concern (Kaye & Wolff, 1997; Berkowitz & Wolff, 2000).

Today, nonprofit organizations of all sorts frequently engage in collaborations with other organizations in their communities (see, for example, the entire Fall 2001 issue of the practice-oriented journal *Nonprofit Quarterly*, which is devoted to this topic). Most nonprofits currently belong to a number of these collaborations. More generally stated, the purposes of these groups are to (1) leverage resources, (2) increase impact, (3) cut costs, (4) coordinate strategy, (5) increase organizational visibility, (6) network, and (7) build the overall capacity of the partnering organizations to deliver services or otherwise respond to community needs.

Funders increasingly are asking for collaborations to support the projects they fund, as evidence of community involvement. Training and technical assistance about how to create and sustain collaborations are offered by nonprofit associations, university management training programs, and management assistance organizations. Numerous journal articles and book chapters on this subject have appeared in the nonprofit management literature over the last 5 years. In short, collaborations are an idea whose time has come.

But any idea whose time has come must also be proven to be effective and worth the scarce resources it uses up. A fundamental question (which has so far been little addressed in evaluation studies of collaborations) is whether the resources used in collaboration have greater impact than if they had been used in separate actions by the participant organizations or community groups. This question is important, because there is always a transaction cost associated with the act of collaboration itself—not only the costs of operating the collaboration, but also the time and effort put into it by the participants. Moreover, no matter how powerful the concept, its implementation can usually be improved. The evaluation of collaborations can provide evidence of outcome and impact and can help improve the process by which the collaboration operates.

The total amount of resources, including dollars and time, invested in collaborative efforts is extensive. Yet, the evaluation of these entities remains sporadic at best, and the results unclear. Kegler, Steckler, McLeroy, and Malek (1998) noted that, "given the major role of coalitions in community health promotion as it is currently practiced in the United States, it is surprising how little is known empirically about this approach" (p. 338). In a recent review of healthy community coalitions in Massachusetts, Berkowitz and Wolff (2000) surveyed 40 coalitions on their evaluation practices. Even though 89% reported involvement in some form of evaluation of their work, these evaluations were "irregular, partial and nonsystematic." Berkowitz and Wolff noted that "very few initiatives took part in regular, formal, planned evaluation over an extended period of time" (p. 3). The experience of these coalitions seems to be representative of coalitions across the country.

Roussos and Fawcett (2000) reviewed 34 studies of 252 collaborative partnerships and concluded that the "findings . . . are insufficient to make strong conclusions about the effects of partnerships on population-based outcomes" (p. 400). In a review of 68 studies of health changes based on collaborative interventions, Kreuter, Lezin, and Young (2000) could find only six examples clearly documenting that change had occurred.

The reviewers suggest that collaborations sometimes simply prove to be inefficient mechanisms for bringing about community change, particularly if they are not carefully planned at the outset (for instance, because collaborations often are poorly resourced, and staffed by volunteers, so they simply do not have the resources needed to match interventions and strategies to long-term outcomes). However, other possibilities are that real systems change often does occur as a result of collaboration activities, but is difficult to measure because of methodological or resource limits on evaluation. Or, finally, that funders and communities may simply have unrealistic expectations about what collaborations can deliver: They may be better suited to bringing diverse groups in a community together, then need to be followed by more intensively structured (and funded) interventions, to create the desired change.

Foster-Fishman et al. (2001), in their review of 80 articles, chapters, and practitioners' guides focused on collaborations, take a different slant on the available literature: They look for elements of a framework that define the core competencies and processes that collaborations need to be successful. Their meta-analysis reveals four main factors: member capacity (the skills and knowledge of individual collaboration members), relational capacity (the climate, vision, and working process of the collaboration), organizational capacity (the leadership, work procedures, communication style, resources, and improvement orientation of the collaboration), and programmatic capacity (the objectives and goals of the collaboration, as they relate to defined community needs). Their focus on collaboration capacity is in keeping with current funder and nonprofit community emphasis on nonprofit organizational capacity building (Backer, 2001b).

The results of such initial reviews and meta-analyses must be seen as a warning to the collaboration movement. This warning suggests that, unless collaborators begin seriously evaluating the outcomes of their work, they will face more questions from funders and critics. Even more important, they will miss opportunities to learn about the process and outcome of collaborations that can be improved. Fortunately, both science-based and wisdom literatures provide guidance for collaboration leaders, funders, and evaluators, in this regard.

This volume explores methods by which collaborations in the human services can be evaluated. This chapter provides an overview of what we mean when we say "collaboration," what the key advantages and challenges of these approaches are, what we mean when we say "evaluation of a collaboration," and some of the associated approaches and challenges. It also offers a brief preview of what is in the rest of this volume.

DEFINITIONS OF COLLABORATION

Briefly defined, a *collaboration* brings together two or more agencies, groups, or organizations at the local, state, or national level, to achieve some common purpose of systems change (Backer & Norman, 1998, 2000). Collaborations involve the sharing of goals, activities, responsibilities, and resources. The relationship can be temporary or permanent, informal or structured through contracts or other legal agreements, and can be very limited or quite broad in scope. However, collaborations maintain the basic legal and fiscal independence of the member organizations. They are usually voluntary, at least in principle (although perhaps not in practice because of requirements of funders or other factors).

The organizational members of collaborations may include nonprofit organizations (e.g., community health or social service providers), grassroots groups, intermediary organizations (such as technical assistance organizations that support or provide training for nonprofit groups in a community), funders (foundation or government), policy-making bodies (city councils, county boards of supervisors, etc.), businesses, public schools, colleges and universities, or professional and trade organizations. The life of the collaboration is often facilitated by meetings of representatives from these member organizations.

Two critical dimensions by which collaborations differ are the degree of formality or informality of their organization and the degree of mutual accountability versus separate accountability in how the organizational members relate to each other. In fact, these two dimensions provide a way by which we can think about how collaborations as a type of social organization contrast with other groups, in the following way:

mutual accountability

                                                                        merger

                                                        joint venture

                                            strategic alliance

informal   **collaboration**   *formal*
organization   *organization*
                               coalition

              committee

     informal network

separate accountability

The boundaries between a collaboration and a coalition, or between other types of organizations in this array, are not fixed precisely. However, for the most part, these seven classes of social organizations (including collaboration at their center) are relatively easy to distinguish, as the following definitions make clear:

- *Informal network:* a deliberately unstructured activity jointly supported by a group of community organizations. These informal networks are often powerful institutions, despite their informal nature, and in part because of it, especially if they are composed of powerful individuals.
- *Committee:* a structured but unincorporated, and usually time-limited-activity, group of people representing their community organizations, getting together for regular meetings to take action together on particular issues.
- *Coalition:* such community-based groups, often focused on policy change or community development goals, are more structured than a committee, but less formal than a partnership/ collaboration. They often come from the grassroots actions of a community to address a problem seen by community members more than by the organized leadership of the community. They often are organized to give more power to groups seen as underrepresented or at least underserved by a public body.
- *Strategic alliance:* a structured, contractual relationship between two or more organizations to accomplish some particular goal, while maintaining the separateness of their individual organizations. These approaches have been increasingly common in the nonprofit world, as they have been for years in the business arena. David LaPiana, of Strategic Solutions, has written extensively about strategic alliances (see *www.lapiana.org* for more details).
- *Joint venture:* a more formally structured legal relationship between the partners, in which there is a commitment of capital resources to accomplish a certain task. Usually, joint ventures are time-limited, and they are always focused on specific activities. However, sometimes they can have an ongoing life, as well, especially if they are very successful.
- *Merger:* legally bringing together two or more organizations with overlapping missions and target audiences, to increase efficiency and mission accomplishment.

There is also a time dimension tied to degree of formality, in that mergers, at least in theory, are permanent arrangements for groups to work together; informal networks or committees are typically not intended to last.

What is most critical for people working in a collaboration (or evaluating it from the outside) is to understand what assumptions members of a particular collaboration are working on in defining their values and operations. How structured is the organization of the collaboration? To what extent is there mutual accountability? Do the members of the collaboration understand the use of this term in somewhat the same way?

There is a potential for trouble if a group uses one term but really means another. A group using the term "partnership," for example, but really meaning "coalition," may be surprised to find that some of its members (and others in the community) may well expect such things as financial disclosure, due diligence, written agreement documents, joint evaluations, and a seat at the board table. One very troubling reason for the failure of mutual efforts is simply this: The parties do not agree on the meaning of the words they use.

In the literature and wisdom knowledge base reviewed in this book, moreover, these distinctions in terms are often not observed. Also, most in the field precisely regard *collaboration* and *partnership* to be interchangeable terms. And some of the science and experience reported here for coalitions also seem to apply quite well to their more structured, mutually accountable cousins. Further debate in the management and behavioral sciences will no doubt be needed to resolve some of the definitional issues raised by the graphic, but it is not the purpose of this volume to do so. We use the term *collaboration* here, because it best reflects the semistructured, somewhat mutually accountable entities being discussed throughout: Some of the discussion and examples may lean a little more toward partnership, and some a little more towards coalition, but this is the general range in which our discourse will take place.

One other source of difficulty lies in another set of terms, used to describe the *process* by which the collaboration operates. People use an immense array of such terms, and adopt a variety of approaches to getting themselves to the table and to agreement. In one recent study (Backer, Howard, & Koone, 2000), 17 grantees used 11 different names to describe the process for their collaborations, for example, "total quality management," "business process engineering," "conflict resolution model," "community decision-making model," "consensus decision-making model," and "interest-based negotiations." Some of these terms reflect well-researched models for systems change adopted by the grantees; others were invented by the grantees, or used rather informally, to designate the process approach they decided to implement. Mediation also provides a process model, which will be discussed further in one of the chapters in this book, concerning the human dynamics of collaborations.

PURPOSE OF THIS VOLUME

This volume originally was commissioned to provide support for grantees and evaluators of the federal Center for Mental Health Services (CMHS) School and Community Action Grant Program (which awards grants to enable collaborations for guiding systems change in youth violence prevention programming, both school- and community-based). This program is similar to another CMHS grant-making program, the Community Action Grant Program, which awards similar grants for systems change related to improved services for severely mentally ill individuals in communities, also emphasizing a collaboration approach.

This volume is intended to be used by the people who create and run community collaborations of various types (but especially those in the health and human service fields), the people who evaluate them, and the people who fund them or live with them in the community. Collaborations in nonprofit arts are described in a recent publication (Backer, 2002), and much of what is presented here also would be useful in evaluating arts and culture collaborations. This volume includes a fair amount of attention to published literature and the wisdom experience of other people who have evaluated or organized collaborations. It is intended to provide practice guidelines for (1) decision making, (2) strategic planning, and (3) whole-community action.

SUCCESSES AND CHALLENGES OF COLLABORATION

Some collaborations clearly have had real impact in guiding systems change— their basic reason for existence—as already described, to design a program or implement it, or to change a policy or procedure. What is being changed is almost always at the systems level within a single organization, a group of them, or an entire community, which is a main part of the reason a group of community entities have to come together to make the change happen.

Backer, Howard, and Koone (2000) report some significant successes in this regard for the first 17 of the Community Action Grant projects (an evaluation of three subsequent groups of these grantees now is under way). For instance, the City of Berkeley's Mental Health Division created an effective community collaboration (involving dozens of participating community agencies and groups), which worked together to implement Assertive Community Treatment for severely mentally ill people in that Northern California community. The resulting program now has more than $1 million in annual funding to provide significant outreach, case management, and related services, to get mentally ill people into treatment and keep them enrolled for as long as recovery takes.

Similar successes of collaborations were reported by Backer (2001a) for a youth violence prevention program funded by a foundation. As of this writing, the School and Community Action Grant program evaluation, also being conducted by Backer, Howard, and Koone, is still in its early stages, so conclusions about success cannot yet be made.

In other cases, collaborations fail to have as much impact as was hoped for. Many are created without first conducting an appropriate *assessment*, by asking questions such as, Is a collaboration the right step at this time, in this community, to address this particular problem? Moreover, few collaborations are created with appropriate attention to the behavioral and management science that has accumulated over the last few years, both about how to create partnerships or collaborations and about how to sustain them over time. As a result, even when collaboration is the right step to take, it may not be realized well, so it does not work or does not last.

The dysfunction and mortality rates among community collaborations are high, not unlike the high divorce rate in American society (Backer & Norman, 1998). Although the types of collaborations highlighted in this volume have important differences from the individual counterpart of marriage (e.g., they typically do not involve comingling of funds), they are similar, in that they involve deeply shared values, common missions that may spread out over a period of time, and emotionally complex relationships that spring from the first two features. Funders, community leaders, and others helping to create collaborations would do well to heed the relevant French proverb, "Marry in haste, repent at leisure." And, in some cases, premarital counseling, in the form of training about how to engage in successful collaboration prior to embarking on one, can be essential to success (Backer & Norman, 2000).

IMPORTANCE OF EVALUATION

To document the successes and challenges, and to understand them so that the collaborations of today, as well as the collaborations of tomorrow, can be improved, evaluation is needed. Some of the specific purposes evaluation can serve are discussed later and in subsequent chapters.

Given the limited empirical knowledge about collaborations that currently exists, individual evaluations and efforts to synthesize their findings are needed, in order to answer fundamental questions about whether the financial and human investments made in collaborations are in fact desirable. For instance, in the two federal grant programs just mentioned, half of the funding awarded is earmarked specifically to support the development and operation of a community collaboration (sometimes a new effort, sometimes one that builds on an existing collaborative group within the community). Is this funding best spent on that collaborative process, or might it instead be used to increase the scope of the actual implementation, based on an award to one grantee who will "go it alone" or make use of whatever threads of partnership already exist in the community?

Collaborations take time, and may introduce uncertainties or conflicts into the process of systems change that might not have existed without them. Sometimes, the leaders of collaborations already know what they want to accomplish and attempt to use the collaborative structure as a way of engineering consent, without considering alternative paths in any serious way. And sometimes groups come to the table of collaboration only interested in meeting their own narrow objectives, without any serious intent to engage in a true partnership for community change.

These problems are amplified when funders require collaborations as a condition of grant support for a systems change effort, without a dialogue with the community to determine whether collaboration is in fact the right path to pursue in achieving a certain set of systems change outcomes. Under such circumstances, participation in the collaboration may be half-hearted at best, and cynical or intentionally sabotaging at worst.

Evaluation will not solve all of these problems or shortcomings of collaborations, of course; nor can the accumulation of evaluation knowledge provide secure paths by which a community or a funder can determine in advance whether a collaboration is the right step to take on the road to systems change. But evaluation can play a role in the accumulation of both scientific knowledge and wisdom about how collaborations contribute to systems change. And the state of evaluation practice can be influenced positively, both by exploring the science on collaboration (which is the subject of the next section of this chapter), and by looking at the issues involved in the evaluation of collaborations (which is the topic of the rest of this volume.).

SCIENCE ABOUT COLLABORATION STRATEGIES

Collaborations have always existed informally in communities (Winer & Ray, 1994), and those that spring from the grassroots are sometimes referred to as "coalitions," for which there is a distinct but highly related literature (Kass & Freudenberg, 1997; LaBonte, 1997; Wandersman, Goodman, &

Butterfoss, 1997). Community collaborations or coalitions have been especially prominent in the public health arena (Butterfoss, Goodman & Wandersman, 1993). For example, in the substance abuse prevention field, more than 250 partnerships, each with multiple public and private groups involved, have been supported by the federal government through the Center for Substance Abuse Prevention (Yin et al., 1997). The Robert Wood Johnson Foundation has, for almost 10 years, funded the "Fighting Back" coalitions in 14 cities. That same foundation also supports "Join Together," a national coordinating center for community substance abuse prevention, which provides technical assistance to coalitions, as does the Community Anti-Drug Coalitions of America organization (Backer & Norman, 2000).

As mentioned, many collaborations are not successful, or at least are not sustained over time, despite continuing need for assistance in creating the systems change they provide. The reasons for this are numerous, according to research on this topic (Backer & Norman, 1998, 2000; Kaye & Wolff, 1997; M. Kreuter, personal communication, Feb. 5, 1998; Kreuter & Lezin, 1998). Turf and competition issues often arise, and there is often "bad history" in the community from past partnerships that have failed. Sometimes, the collaboration becomes more interested in sustaining itself than in doing the work it was originally created to do. And many such groups have endless planning meetings that do not lead to action. The size of the collaboration also may have a bearing on its style and method of operations: Large, community-wide efforts have many complexities, which, if not carefully managed, can limit their effectiveness.

There is, as a result, some skepticism about the current fervor for collaborations, both in the literature on this subject and among those involved in such activities in communities. Former Surgeon General Jocelyn Elders put it humorously, but pointedly, in an address to the Rosalynn Carter Mental Health Symposium several years ago:

> Collaboration has been defined as an unnatural act between non-consenting adults. We all say we want to collaborate, but what we really mean is that we want to continue doing things as we have always done them while others change to fit what we are doing. (Backer & Norman, 1998, p. 7)

Organized practice and science on this subject are little used to guide the creation and sustaining of collaborations. Strategies for creating and sustaining community collaborations and partnerships have been studied in education (John S. and James L. Knight Foundation, 1996; Kochar & Erickson, 1993; Tushnet, 1993), mental health (Center for Improving Mental Health Systems,

1995), health communication (Backer & Rogers, 1993), and other fields (Kaye & Wolff, 1997; Mattessich & Monsey, 1992; Schneider, 1994).

Backer and Rogers (1993) draw attention to the management science literatures of interorganizational networking and strategic alliances (Gage & Mandell, 1990; Tichy, 1984), in which considerable empirical research has identified principles for beginning and sustaining partnership-like arrangements. In the business world, major conferences and management magazine articles on strategic alliances are commonplace. This literature has seldom been used in the creation of nonprofit collaborations, however, even though the two types of activity appear to have much in common.

Mattessich and Monsey (1992) reviewed the research literature on collaboration in health, social science, education, and public affairs, and they identified a total of 19 factors from 133 studies examined. These 19 factors, divided below by specific characteristics, provide a good synthesis of critical factors in successful collaboration, supported in large measure by subsequent studies:

Environmental Characteristics

- History of collaboration or cooperation in the community
- Partnership entity seen as a leader in the community
- Political/social climate is favorable

Membership Characteristics

- Mutual respect, understanding, and trust among the members
- Appropriate cross-section of members
- Members see collaboration as in their self-interest
- Ability to compromise

Process/Structure Characteristics

- Members share a stake in both process and outcome
- Multiple layers of decision making
- Flexibility
- Clear roles and policy guidelines are developed
- Adaptability

Communication Characteristics

- Open and frequent communication
- Established informal and formal communication links

Purpose Characteristics

- Concrete, attainable goals and objectives
- Shared vision
- Unique purpose

Resource Characteristics

- Sufficient funds
- A skilled convener

Some research now is being conducted on the training and resource infrastructure that supports collaboration development. For instance, under funding support from the Stuart Foundation, Floyd Brown of the University of Washington has surveyed California and Washington community partnerships, to determine what kinds of training and technical assistance they have received, and how successful these interventions have been (Brown, 1998).

Funders are beginning to explore both the strengths and limits of collaborations, with recent essays in the philanthropic literature. For example, Kitzi (1997), in a *Foundation News and Commentary* article on partnerships, reflects that most foundations find it easier to require partnerships among their grantees than to create them within philanthropy. The McKnight Foundation (1991) offered the following well-balanced commentary on partnerships for an initiative to help families in poverty:

> Collaboration results in easier, faster and more coherent access to services and benefits and in greater effects on systems. Working together is not a substitute for adequate funding, although the synergistic effects of the collaborating partners often result in creative ways to overcome obstacles. (p. 2)

In the health arena, collaborations are also the focus of considerable attention. In a critical review of the literature, Kreuter and Lezin (1998) conclude that collaborations can be effective in changing health status and health systems, but only under certain tightly specified conditions. They cite six programs in which such health systems change occurred.

Bibeau et al. (1996) found that a community coalition was instrumental in increasing the ability of a local clinic to provide health services to the poor. Schacht (1998), in a study for the California Wellness Foundation, evaluated grants made to community collaborations of county health clinics, which, in turn, gave grants to individual clinics and supported association-wide infrastructure development. Using these partnerships as intermediaries for a grant-making program generally seemed to be successful. In two cases, the grant making actually helped develop a partnership in a county that did not have one before (and there were many challenges in getting the 60 health clinics in Los Angeles County to come together for this purpose). The evaluation found that stronger infrastructure boosts clinic productivity, so there were direct health outcomes from this program as well.

DEFINITIONS OF EVALUATION

Many of the foregoing discussions of collaborations and partnerships do not even refer to systematic evaluation of these efforts, because there often is none. Subjective impressions of policy makers, funders, and community leaders, plus the continuing enthusiasm of participants for being part of the collaboration and keeping it moving, are the evaluative measures that count. However, as collaborations have become more extensive, more central to the achievement of important community goals, and a greater object of funder attention, a greater likelihood of evaluation emerges. Collaboration members and the funders of these entities, therefore, have increased needs for information and guidance about the complexities of evaluation. These are addressed throughout this volume.

As in the traditional program evaluation literature, evaluations of collaborations tend to be of two kinds: *process* (in which the emphasis is on gathering data about how the collaboration functions and how it might be improved over time) and *outcome* (measuring to what extent the collaboration empirically meets its objectives and, in only a few cases, what impact its interventions have on identified target audiences or the community as a whole). In addition, evaluation of collaborations can be defined in terms of who does them: *self-evaluation* by the collaboration staff or members themselves; and *external evaluation*—usually that required by a funder. The external evaluation sometimes is commissioned (and to some extent controlled, thus raising questions about its objectivity) by the collaboration, and sometimes by the funder.

SCIENCE ABOUT EVALUATION OF COLLABORATIONS

As already mentioned, in the most comprehensive review of collaborations in health to date, Roussos and Fawcett (2000) report that collaborations have become increasingly popular strategies for community health improvement, but only limited empirical evidence of their impact has been gathered to date. Their review, based on 34 studies of collaboration process and outcomes, reinforces the importance of evaluation and of stakeholder involvement in evaluation strategy. It also identifies some larger context variables that evaluators need to consider in designing and carrying out evaluations of collaborations:

- Community social and economic factors
- Social capital
- Context in which the collaboration was created and in which it operates
- Community control in agenda setting

Florin, Mitchell, and Stevenson (1993) report a methodology for measuring the training and technical assistance needs of community-based partnerships. Fawcett et al. (1997); Francisco, Paine, and Fawcett (1993); Gabriel (2000); and Gillies (1997) all present methods for monitoring and evaluating health partnerships. Collaboration strategies, their impact, and ways of measuring that impact also have been discussed in the healthy communities movement (Minkler, 1997). Francisco et al. (2001) described an on-line Community Tool Box, which includes approaches and instruments specific to evaluation of community collaboration.

Fawcett et al. (1993) have developed a model for evaluation, which emerged from the work of the Work Group on Health Promotion and Community Development at the University of Kansas (see chapter 5). It assumes that collaborations are evaluated in order to understand and improve their process (the pattern of actions taken to bring about change), outcome (changes in community policies, programs, and practices), and impact (actual changes in community-level indicators of individual behavior or community quality of life). Evaluation data are collected to address five key questions:

- Was the community in fact mobilized through the collaboration?
- What changes in the community resulted from the collaboration?
- Is there a change in reported individual behavior of target audiences?
- Is there a change in reported behavior of the community as a whole?
- Is there a change in the quality of life or functioning of the community overall?

Fifteen evaluative measures are taken under this model, ranging from members participating in the collaboration, to goals of the collaboration, to community-level indicators of impact (e.g., for an alcohol-oriented collaboration, archival records of single-nighttime vehicle crashes). The model was tested on Project Freedom, a community substance abuse prevention collaboration in Wichita, Kansas.

Gabriel (2000) presents some of the challenges evaluators face in working with collaborations:

- An ever-changing array of interventions
- Difficulty in specifying the target populations precisely
- The unavailability of traditional no-treatment control groups
- Poor, or at least underspecified, connections between the immediate outcomes of the intervention the collaboration is promoting, and the ultimately desired impact

One potentially useful framework for thinking about some of these complexities is provided by Yin et al. (1997), in their work on the federal Center for Substance Abuse Prevention's Community Prevention Partnerships evaluation. The Community Partnership Evaluation Framework has eight collaboration variables, which have been generalized for presentation here:

- Characteristics
- Capacity
- Community actions
- Immediate process and activity outcomes
- Target population outcomes
- Community outcomes
- Target population and community impacts
- Contextual conditions

Yin and Ware (2000) discuss some of the options for using both archival and survey data concerning substance abuse, to develop evaluation research designs. The strategies they outline could readily be adapted to other fields.

ABOUT THIS VOLUME

This volume has five main themes, each of which is addressed by a chapter:

- Multicultural dimensions of collaborations and how to deal with them (chapter 2, Norman)

- Human dynamics associated with evaluation of collaborations and how to handle them (chapter 3, Backer & Kunz)
- Instruments and other resources for evaluating collaborations, including an appendix of worksheets (chapter 4, Wolff)
- Approaches to interpreting results of collaborative evaluations and to evaluating the whole community's involvement with a collaboration (chapter 5, Francisco, Schultz, & Fawcett)
- Evaluating collaborations in a specific subject, youth violence prevention at the community level (chapter 6, Guerra)

There are also two brief pieces to set these chapters in context: a foreword by a leader in empowerment evaluation (Wandersman) and a commentary by a funder (Bare). Taken together, these discussions of how to plan, conduct, report on, and use results from the evaluation of a collaboration can help collaboration members, other community leaders, funders, and evaluators themselves address the complex tasks discussed here.

ACKNOWLEDGMENT

The author acknowledges the helpful conceptual and editorial input of Elizabeth Howard, Human Interaction Research Institute, to the development of this chapter.

REFERENCES

Backer, T. E. (2001a). *Cross-site evaluation for the planning phase of Knight Foundation's Initiative to Promote Youth Development and Prevent Youth Violence.* Encino, CA: Human Interaction Research Institute.

Backer, T. E. (2001b). Strengthening nonprofits: Foundation initiatives for capacity building. In C. J. DeVita & C. Fleming (Eds.), *Building capacity in nonprofit organizations* (pp. 31–83). Washington, DC: Urban Institute.

Backer, T. E. (2002). *Partnership as an art form: What works and what doesn't in nonprofit arts partnerships.* Encino, CA: Human Interaction Research Institute.

Backer, T. E., Howard, E. A., & Koone, U. S. (2000). *Final report: Evaluation of the Community Action Grant program — Phase 1: Round 1 grantees.* Encino, CA: Human Interaction Research Institute.

Backer, T. E., & Norman, A. (1998). *Best practices in multicultural coalitions: Phase I report to the California Endowment.* Northridge, CA: Human Interaction Research Institute.

Backer, T. E., & Norman, A. J. (2000). Partnerships and community change. *California Politics and Policy,* 39–44.

Backer, T. E., & Rogers, E. M. (Eds.). (1993). *Organizational aspects of health communication campaigns: What works?* Newbury Park, CA: Sage.

Berkowitz, B., & Wolff, T. (2000). *The spirit of the coalition.* Washington, DC: American Public Health Association.

Bibeau, D. L., et al. (1996). The role of a community coalition in the development of health services for the poor and uninsured. *International Journal of Health Services, 26*(1), 93–110.

Brown, F. (1998). Personal communication, February 22.

Butterfoss, F., Goodman, R., & Wandersman, A. (1993). Community coalitions for prevention and health promotion. *Health Education Research, 8*(3), 315–330.

Center for Improving Mental Health Systems. (1995). *Training manual: New Mexico Partnerships for Systems Improvement.* Northridge, CA: Human Interaction Research Institute.

Fawcett, S. B., et al. (1993). *Work group evaluation handbook: Evaluating and supporting community initiatives for health and development.* Lawrence, KS: Work Group on Health Promotion and Community Development, The University of Kansas.

Florin, P., Mitchell, R., & Stevenson, J. (1993). Identifying training and technical assistance needs in community coalitions: A developmental approach. *Health Education Research, 8*(3), 417–432.

Foster-Fishman, P. G., et al. (2001). Building collaborative capacity in community coalitions: A review and integrative framework. *American Journal of Community Psychology, 29*(2), 241–261.

Francisco, V. T., et al. (2001). Using internet-based resources to build community capacity: The Community Tool Box. *American Journal of Community Psychology, 29*(2), 293–299.

Francisco, V. T., Paine, A. L., & Fawcett, S. B. (1993). A methodology for monitoring and evaluating community health coalitions. *Health Education Research, 8*(3), 403–416.

Gabriel, R. (2000). Methodological challenges in evaluating community partnerships & coalitions: Still crazy after all these years. *Journal of Community Psychology, 28*(3), 339–352.

Gage, R. W., & Mandell, M. P. (Eds.). (1990). *Strategies for managing intergovernmental policies and networks.* New York: Praeger.

Gillies, P. (1997). *The effectiveness of alliances and partnerships for health promotion.* Conference working paper, Fourth International Conference on Health Promotion, Jakarta, Indonesia.

John S. & James L. Knight Foundation (1996). *Learning to collaborate: Lessons from School—College Partnerships in the Excellence in Education Program.* Miami: Author.

Kass, D., & Freudenberg, N. (1997). Coalition building to prevent childhood lead poisoning: A case study from New York City. In M. Minkler (Ed.), *Community organizing and community building for health* (pp. 278–290). New Brunswick, NJ: Rutgers University Press.

Kaye, G., & Wolff, T. (1997). *From the ground up: A workbook on coalition building and community development.* Amherst, MA: AHEC/Community Partners.

Kegler, M., Steckler, A., McLeroy, K., & Malek, S. (1998). Factors that contribute to effective community health promotion coalitions: A study of 10 Project ASSIST coalitions in North Carolina. *Health Education and Behavior, 25,* 338–353.

Kitzi, J. (1997, March/April). Easier said than done. *Foundation News and Commentary*, 39–41.

Kochar, C., & Erickson, M. R. (1993). *Business-education partnerships for the 21st century: A practical guide for school improvement*. Gaithersburg, MD: Aspen.

Kreuter, M., & Lezin, N. (1998). *Are consortia/collaboratives effective in changing health status and health systems?* Atlanta: Health 2000.

Kreuter, M. W., Lezin, N. A., & Young, L. A. (2000). Evaluating community-based collaborative mechanisms: Implications for practitioners. *Health Promotion Practice, 1*(1), 49–63.

Labonte, R. (1997). Community, community development and the forming of authentic partnerships: Some critical reflections. In M. Minkler (Ed.), *Community organizing and community building for health* (pp. 122–145). New Brunswick, NJ: Rutgers University Press.

Mattessich, P. W., & Monsey, B. R. (1992). *Collaboration: What makes it work*. St. Paul, MN: Amherst H. Wilder Foundation.

McKnight Foundation. (1991). *The Aid to Families in Poverty Program*. Minneapolis: Author.

Minkler, M. (Ed.). *Community organizing and community building for health*. New Brunswick, NJ: Rutgers University Press.

Roussos, S. T., & Fawcett, S. B. (2000). A review of collaborative partnerships as a strategy for improving community health. *Annual Review of Public Health, 21,* 369–402.

Schacht, J. (1998). Creating partnerships with clinic associations to preserve the safety net. *Health Affairs, 17*(1), 248–252.

Schneider, A. (1994). Building strategic alliances. *New Designs for Youth Development, 11*(3), 23–26.

Tichy, N. M. (1984). Networks in organizations. In P. C. Nystrum & W. H. Starbuck (Eds.), *Handbook of organizational design* (Vol. 2, pp. 223–267). Oxford: Oxford University Press.

Tushnet, N. (1993). *A guide to developing educational partnerships*. Washington, DC: U.S. Department of Education, Office of Educational Research and Improvement.

Wandersman, A., Goodman, R. M., & Butterfoss, F. D. (1997). Understanding coalitions and how they operate: An "open systems" organizational framework. In M. Minkler (Ed.), *Community organizing and community building for health* (pp. 261–277). New Brunswick, NJ: Rutgers University Press.

Winer, M., & Ray, K. (1994). *Collaboration handbook: Creating, sustaining and enjoying the journey*. St. Paul, MN: Amherst H. Wilder Foundation.

Yin, R. K., & Ware, A. I. (2000). Using outcome data to evaluate community drug prevention initiatives: Pushing the state-of-the-art. *American Journal of Community Psychology, 28*(3), 323–338.

Yin, R. K., et al. (1997). Outcomes from CSAP's community partnership program: Findings from the national cross-site evaluation. *Evaluation and Program Planning, 20*(3), 345–355.

CHAPTER 2

Multicultural Issues in Collaboration: Some Implications for Multirater Evaluation

Alex J. Norman

There are many models of collaboration currently being used to achieve a more coordinated approach to providing integrated services to various needy populations. As examples, there are public–private partnerships, coalitions, alliances, and interagency collaborations that operate through memoranda of understanding or letters of cooperation. The implications for evaluation discussed later in the chapter apply to all of those models or approaches in which the participants in the process come from different cultural or ethnic groups. For purposes of the discussion that follows, *collaboration* is defined as "a fluid process through which diverse, autonomous actors (organizations or individuals) undertake a joint initiative, solve shared problems, or otherwise achieve common goals" (Abramson & Rosenthal, 1995).

This chapter presents some general issues that should be considered when evaluating collaborations across cultures, and is based on the author's practice experience and observations as a facilitator and consultant to organizations and community-based collaborations (i.e., school–community, public–private, public–public, interdisciplinary, and interagency). General issues are discussed first, followed by cultural issues that have implications for evaluation at the planning, implementation, and maintenance phases of the collaborations. The reader should be cautioned that these are not exhaustive lists of issues, but ones that seem to be most pressing. As we gain more experience in collaborating across cultures, we will also develop more knowledge about the importance of other issues.

The first issue that must be considered is that collaborations are not organizations per se. That is to say, they are not put together as orderly, functional wholes in the way that traditional organizations are. They are "virtual organizations" in the sense that, although there may be a group of individuals or a combination of organizational representatives and individuals who make up the collaboration, there is often an absence of an infrastructure that is characteristic of a traditional organization. Frequently, there is not staff that can be readily called upon to take action or carry out orders. There is no board with responsibility to create and monitor policies. The dotted-line relationships do not carry with them a direct accountability or reporting responsibility and frequently allow issues to fall between the cracks.

The individual stakeholders who make up the collaboration more often have primary duties or responsibilities that direct their loyalties (and much of their energies) elsewhere. Many of the actions of participants in collaborations are directed toward "What's in it for me or my agency?" and not "What is the best action to achieve the collaborative goals?" In situations such as these, a more passive approach is likely to be assumed, until an issue directly affecting the individual or their specific agency is discussed. Consequently, a traditional approach to evaluation is likely to miss the mark, because it is not designed to fit the collaboration process, but rather is an overlay of a model used to evaluate programs or projects that are operated by traditional organizations that have traditional, direct-reporting relationships with their staffs.

Another important issue to be addressed is that many of the participants in the collaboration often come from organizations that have a history of competing for the same resources. This competitive history is difficult to overcome, because the organizational representatives who are asked to be less competitive and more cooperative in the collaboration are home-based in their competitive environments. A lack of trust may be present, which prevents an actual collaboration from happening. Often, in its stead are meetings in which stakeholders may come together for networking—exchanging information for their own benefit—but with little concerted behavior or shared effort taking place.

In such situations, what might be evaluated is not a collaboration, but rather a networking group of individuals exchanging information and ideas.

Therefore, an evaluation model that seeks to measure the effectiveness of a collaboration must ensure that collaborative behaviors, not individual or agency-centered behaviors, are being addressed.

Such a situation involving these issues occurred while the author was a consultant with the Los Angeles Children's Planning Council (CPC), a quasi-public–private partnership designed to improve coordination of services to children and families in Los Angeles County. The CPC divided the county into eight Service Planning Areas, creating virtual organizations of representatives of agencies, institutions, and individuals, with CPC providing staff liaison services and a small grant ($40,000) to be used for clerical support and to defray operating expenses.

In one Service Planning Area with the greatest needs and fewest resources, the two cofacilitators, who had a history of being competitive with each other, held major responsibilities in other organizations and were often pressured by their primary jobs to devote their energies elsewhere. The combination of their competitiveness and the pressures for their time used a tremendous amount of energy to resolve interpersonal or agency-centered issues. Consequently, some tasks simply did not get done, because of work overload or, as one cofacilitator expressed it, "doing the jobs we are paid to do." It was not uncommon for the facilitators to remind the county liaison that, unlike county staff, they were not being paid to attend the various meetings called by CPC. Others who were given committee assignments voiced similar frustrations.

A major implication for those seeking to evaluate collaborations is that the model or approach be crafted to fit the specific collaboration goals or objectives, and that the actions of the collaborators be directed toward the active performance of behaviors that will support the goals and objectives. Thus, the actors in the collaboration must play a more active role in the identification and appraisal of evaluation criteria.

CULTURAL ISSUES

In a study conducted for the California Endowment, Backer and Norman (1998) identified 13 factors that contributed to the success of multicultural coalitions:

- Efforts by coalition leadership to plan ahead for sustainability
- Creation of a process for setting and communicating shared goals
- Early implementation of strategies for managing conflict

- Implementation of strategies for handling cultural stereotypes
- Understanding of the change process by coalition leadership
- Use of volunteer structures that are nonthreatening to other agencies
- Having a supportive lead agency that may serve as a fiscal agent
- Development of a written strategic plan for coalition operations
- Orientation by coalition leadership to a basic vision
- Evolution of greater formality, if the coalition is to implement programs
- Acknowledging poverty as a central issue underlying problems
- Use of ties that a coalition has to related organizations
- Building social capital in communities, through coalition activities

There were five challenges that the successful coalitions had to overcome: (1) a mistrust of the collaborative process itself; (2) bad history from participating in previous coalitions in the same community; (3) becoming more concerned with perpetuating the coalition, rather than addressing the issues for which it was formed; (4) being the product of a top-down, rather than a bottom-up, creation; and (5) difficulties in recruiting staff able to work within a coalition structure.

Although it is difficult to pinpoint the most pressing issue in cross-cultural collaborations, the one issue that surfaces most is that of a lack of trust of the institutions and the institutional representatives by members of cultural or ethnic minority group members (Norman, 1996). For example, in 1996, three major on-campus fights with racial and gang overtones, during a 4-year period, prompted the city council and the Palm Springs School District to form a broad-based community collaboration of representatives of the school, the student body, the city, community individuals, and organizations, to determine the root causes and to make recommendations for action. This Intergroup Relations Committee met 23 times over a 13-month period, holding public hearings, committee meetings, and strategy sessions. They issued a 32-page report that identified the root causes as "class and socioeconomic differences and an insufficient community response." With much fanfare, they recommended that a community-wide strategy be used to address the issues, similar to the approach used to develop the report.

After months of delay, and no action during the summer, the school district pursued its own strategy, and the city viewed the issues as "school-based." Despite appeals to the city council, and community efforts to initiate collaborative action, the issue was treated as school-based and therefore as requiring a school response. This approach was counter to that expressed in the Intergroup Relations Study Committee report. However, the power and status groups in the collaboration were the school district and the city council. Thus, an already untrusting community became even more untrusting as a result of these actions on the part of the school district and the city council.

This lack of trust may be the result of an institution's reluctance to share or divulge information that affects people in the community, resistance to open their decision-making process to community participation, or a general lack of familiarity with the institution's way of operating. Regardless of the reason, this lack of trust can manifest itself in the form of verbal attacks or hostile responses, to overtures by representatives of the institution, from community representatives, who may already be suspicious of evaluations. The lack of trust may be carried over to the person(s) conducting the evaluation, who are perceived as representing either the sponsoring institution or funding organization.

Another issue of importance is the possible perception of an unequal balance of power among the collaborators, because of gender, ethnicity, race, culture, or language proficiency. This is not to deny that an unequal balance of power may also result from the status of professions or the size of organizations involved in the collaboration, or other issues (for examples, see Abramson & Rosenthal, 1995). It simply suggests that collaborations, particularly in urban communities, need to include people who might not have experience in dialogue and political debate or who simply might not have a good command of the English language, yet are essential to the collaboration.

The implication for evaluation here is that participation or "creating stakeholders among all participants" becomes a criterion to be considered in the collaboration process (Backer & Norman, 2000). As an example, the City of Long Beach in Los Angeles County has attempted to address this issue by having simultaneous translations during the course of large meetings and collaborations, sometimes conducting three continuous translations. This has greatly increased the level of understanding of issues by participants and increased their tendency to engage in discussions, thereby enriching the collaboration. Beyond those benefits, simultaneous translations have eliminated the restlessness and anger of participants so often experienced in post hoc translations.

The third and final issue I will mention here is that of intergroup conflict, which could have as its base ethnicity, culture, race, or any of the characteristics previously mentioned. It may be labeled "ethnic politics," "gender politics," and so on, but the results are the same: a restraint on the collaboration process, because of the dominance of the representatives of one group over another or, worse still, the end of the collaboration effort (e.g., see Backer & Norman, 1998, 2000). The implication and the challenge for evaluation is that of proposing a model or approach, taking these issues into consideration, but not compromising the collaboration itself.

IMPLICATIONS FOR EVALUATION

When one considers all of the issues mentioned above, the challenge for a successful evaluation might seem enormous but not impossible. Some evaluation approaches focus on developing partnerships at the community level and placing representatives from the community on the evaluation team. Although these types of approaches have lessened hostile feelings toward institutions, increased community representatives' understanding of the evaluation process, or decreased the levels of mistrust, they still are traditional approaches to evaluating nontraditional phenomena. One might argue that these approaches result in a transfer of skills from the evaluation team to the community through its representatives, but they do not create an approach more suitable for evaluating collaborative efforts.

Another approach has been to have community representatives confer with the funding agency regarding a list of acceptable evaluators, based on their credibility and sensitivity to community issues. However, the evaluators, even if selected from among the participating ethnic or cultural groups, continue to employ traditional evaluation methods. So "ethnics evaluating ethnics" does not provide a solution to applying traditional methods to nontraditional phenomena. What I believe the situation calls for is a more collaborative evaluative approach, based on participation of the collaborators in the evaluation scheme, including the negotiation process, to determine the criteria and participation in the appraisal process itself, whether it is designed for evaluative or developmental purposes. Such an approach provides an environment in which the stakeholders, as equal partners in the collaboration, are empowered because they play an active role in determining the content of the collaboration, as well as in the evaluation.

I argue that, in order to successfully evaluate collaborations, from the start we must take into consideration the issues that are likely to result in successful collaborations. Abramson and Rosenthal (1995), Backer and Norman (2000), and Lewis (2001), all have suggested that, in order for collaborations to be successful, issues (i.e., trust, mistrust, etc.) must be acknowledged and dealt with at the formation or planning stage, to create a shared vision or mission; communication must be open and clear. Also, issues of conflict (i.e., ethnic and gender stereotypes, etc.) must be dealt with at the implementation stage. And leadership, power, and participation issues (i.e., ethnic politics, language proficiency, etc.) must be resolved at the maintenance stage, as ongoing tasks.

The complexity of these issues at various stages requires a performance-based approach to evaluation, which can incorporate and accommodate these issues in the process of the development of the collaboration over time—one that can foster more effective communication, increased trust, and increased morale and satisfaction among the collaborators themselves. One such approach, first identified by Bernadin and Beatty (1987), is discussed in the following section.

MULTIRATER FEEDBACK APPROACH TO EVALUATION AND DEVELOPMENT

The contemporary model best suited for evaluating collaborations has been widely used in private sector, corporate organizations, for multiple reasons: as a means for development, as an evaluation tool, as a selection of managerial talent, and as an intervention for organizational change (Tornow, 1993). The approach is referred to in various ways: as 360-degree feedback (Nowack, 1993), as self-assessment and rater-assessment (Harris & Schaubroeck, 1988; Nowack, 1993), and as multirater feedback (Lorsch & Goodearle, 1994). For purposes of this discussion, the term *multirater feedback* will be used.

Multirater feedback is a method of collecting information about a person's work behavior (or performance) from those who work closely with the person (colleagues, coworkers, stakeholders, bosses, etc.). It grew out of an increasing knowledge that "boss-only" feedback about job performance was mostly ineffective in team-oriented environments, which tended to be flattened and collaborative, rather than hierarchal. It was also given impetus when organizations became more customer- or client-oriented and sought to increase employee and consumer involvement in decision making.

For instance, the Hughes Corporation, located in Los Angeles County, incorporated multirater feedback into its Advanced Leadership Program, a multiyear change strategy to move from a space and defense organization to a commercial enterprise. The strategy involved collaborations between the top three levels of management and the peers and external stakeholders at each level. Prior to doing so, the human resource department conducted a study of the literature on multirater feedback as it was used in the industry. This study found that acceptance of multirater feedback ratings is higher than for traditional single-source feedback (Harris & Schaubroeck, 1988; Latham & Wexley, 1982). Also, information from multiple raters tends to be more accurate and to produce a more complete picture of the person's behavior than single-source feedback. The literature study also determined that effectively administered multirater feedback has been shown to foster more effective communication, increased trust, and increased morale and satisfaction between managers and others (Bernadin & Beatty, 1987).

The Hughes human resources department administered questionnaires to 55 managers who had been rated and 132 employees who had been raters. They also conducted focus group discussions with 37 employees and managers who had participated in the study. Brief summaries of some of their findings, which support the collaborative process, are:

- Almost 90% of the employees reported that they could be honest in their responses, and more than 80% felt that their answers would remain confidential.
- More than 75% of the managers reported satisfaction with their involvement with the multirater feedback approach, and a majority (66%) indicated a positive response to using the approach as a part of their performance appraisal.
- A majority of the managers (66%) reported making changes in their behavior as a result of multirater feedback.

These experiences from the corporate sector also address the issues of skepticism, which community collaborators have toward institutions and toward traditional evaluators (who have tended to be white and not persons of color). Even when the evaluators are persons of color, the results of the evaluation and the use of the data are often contentious. The acceptance of the feedback and the accuracy of the information might well overcome those tendencies among collaborators and partners at the community level, who have usually viewed with suspicion the intentions of public institutions and bureaucratic officials.

The most pressing issue that surfaces is a lack of trust, or mistrust, of the institutions with which professionals and nonprofessionals must deal. One reason collaborators have not fared well in many communities is the secretive nature in which information is handled, or the manner in which decisions are made. But there are approaches, such as multirater feedback, which can address the problem.

In multirater feedback, the very factors contributing to improved communication and building trust (e.g., honest responses, satisfaction with involvement, willingness to change behavior) appear to have been an outgrowth of wide participation in the collaborative effort. These results were further emphasized in the Hughes experience, when a content analysis of the open-ended questions revealed that managers and employees perceived that there was an improvement in their communication and involvement, as a result of multirater feedback.

An additional benefit, especially for community partnerships for change, lies in reported improvements in planning and goal-setting, as a result of multirater feedback, while staff indicated an improvement in their leadership skills. When one considers that one of the challenges to successful collaborations is the perpetuation of the collaboration, rather than the goals for which it was formed, this is an important finding. It suggests that, through the multirater process, participants become better at setting goals and are more focused in their vision. Such behaviors are assets for collaborations, particularly when delicate community issues are concerned.

Consequently, it appears that this model can be used to evaluate the success of the collaboration and, at the same time, have a positive influence on developing a team-oriented approach. Certainly, the issues of trust, communication, and power seem to be addressed in the findings just reviewed. Can it work in public sector organizations or public–private partnerships? The author believes it can, if properly applied.

APPLYING MECHANICS OF THE MODEL

The development and implementation of an effective multirater feedback process is complex. It demands that, at each stage in the process—formation, implementation, and maintenance—goals and objectives must be specifically delineated in measurable performance behaviors as they provide the content for collaboration. For example, in the formation stage, in which shared mission and goals are established, along with ground rules for collaborative interaction, the funding organization must be clear about why it is introducing multirater feedback processes into the collaboration. Is the purpose to develop the collaboration or to evaluate the collaborative efforts? Purpose is very important as a guideline for assessing the effectiveness (development) of the collaboration against some intended outcome (evaluation). Thus, the first step is to determine whether multirater feedback is being used strictly as a developmental tool, as part of performance evaluation, or as some combination of both.

Some authors suggest that any multirater feedback process should be introduced as a tool for development, even if it is ultimately to be used as an evaluation methodology (Lorsch & Goodearle, 1994). This is a foreign method to most employees and creates anxiety in both those being rated and those doing the rating, when they learn that their work performance is being evaluated. Although the model engenders trust in the long run, because trust in this type of system is slowly built, it can cause the ratings to be less reliable. Besides, the tendency to rate honestly is fostered when the raters know that no evaluative decisions (such as about pay and promotions) are being made, based on the ratings they provide. These issues suggest that it might be best to begin with the use of multirater feedback in a developmental context, even though later, in its implementation, it may be used as an evaluative tool.

As an example, if the collaboration is a public–private partnership involving a school site and a community organization as colead agencies, and there are other community collaborators, the funding agency should negotiate with representatives of the lead organizations regarding a consensus on the mission and goals of the collaboration in an action planning session. The evaluator(s) should be present from the beginning of the planning and goal-setting process, to help translate the goals into measurable performance behaviors at the operations level. The intended results are clear expectations of the major collaborators in the development of measurable performance behaviors to be acted upon for the funding agency, the colead agencies, and the evaluator.

One implication for the evaluator is that, in addition to having skills as a methodological expert, they must also bring additional skills as a facilitator and, possibly, as a conflict manager. There are further implications for the education and training of evaluative researchers, in terms of the multiple skills needed to be effective in this new environment. Evaluators will need training in human interactive skills, to complement their skills as experts on methodology.

The same types of activity must be duplicated in the formation stage of the collaboration. That is to say, all participants who play an active role in the collaboration should engage in discussions that result in the developing of shared goals and objectives that can be reduced to measurable performance behaviors with the representatives of the colead agencies and the evaluator. This is particularly important, because, once the action planning and goal setting have been completed, the next stage is implementation, when difficulties in communication and interpersonal problems may be the result of previous competitive relationships between the prospective collaborators, or may be the result of limited language proficiency of some of the collaborators, or some other reason.

In any case, even the least powerful voices should have an equal say in determining what specific behaviors, if carried out collaboratively, will lead to goal attainment or achievement of the objectives. Modeling of participation and involvement of the parties to the collaboration must continue, for this is how stakeholders are created and retained. Otherwise, the more powerful voices dominate and chase potential stakeholders away.

At each stage of development, this process of negotiating and developing specific, measurable performance behaviors (with the evaluator as an active collaborator) are necessary, especially at the maintenance stage. At this stage, issues of power and leadership are likely to arise. By having measurable performance behaviors providing the content for all collaborators at all stages of development, all actors will have an active role that they and others can easily observe. Thus, all collaborators must share in the consensus—not just those collaborators from the larger organizations or those persons with the most professional status or those persons who are more politically astute, but every individual who is party to the collaboration.

Also at the maintenance stage, ethnic politics are likely to enter the collaboration, as was the case in the aftermath of the 1992 riots with the Latino/ Black Round Table of Los Angeles, an education-based collaboration of professional and community leaders. In that case, representatives of both factions of the group were hesitant to act, for fear of how they would be viewed in their respective communities. The result was that, by its inaction, the group lost its County Human Relations Commission sponsorship and dissolved shortly thereafter. The school district and community-at-large were deprived of valuable resources at a critical time.

A similar fate happened in the case of the Black–Korean Alliance, established to ease tensions and increase understanding between residents of the African American and Korean American communities. Although there had been prior agreement between the two leaderships to speak with one voice on divisive issues or at critical times, neither group could overcome the pressure of how its members might be perceived as "compromisers" or "sell-outs" in their respective communities. The results were the same—loss of sponsorship by the County Human Relations Unit and dissolution of the collaboration—once again depriving the community of valuable resources at the most critical time of need. In neither of these two cases were the power issues or the stereotypes each group held of the other brought out in open discussion, processed, managed, or resolved.

Therefore, in order to avoid calamities of these kinds, issues of conflict between collaborators and cultural issues between ethnic groups must be "hashed out," because it is just these types of issues that can threaten the solidarity of the collaboration or coalition. Had the collaborators in each of these situations reached consensus about the specific behaviors they were to perform in the planning, implementation, and maintenance stages of their collaboration, possibly their development would have continued, and both end results could have been avoided.

RATING THE RATERS

Once goals and objectives have been operationalized into desired, measurable performance behaviors, each group of collaborators will have a set of performance behaviors attributed to them that they can share with each other. This will build accountability into the system, in that all of the participants in the collaboration will have a complete set of performance behaviors that are linked to their goals and objectives. This is necessary for the collaboration to be successful.

Using a Likert-type scale applied to each performance behavior, the collaborators are in a position to periodically assess or appraise their own performance and the performance of other collaborators with whom they interact. That is, the funding agency can self-assess its performance, as well as assess the performance of the colead agencies; the colead agencies can self-assess their performance, the performance of the funding agency, and the community collaborators; the community collaborators can self-assess their performance, the performance of the colead agencies, and of their colleagues.

The objective of periodic assessments (i.e., quarterly or semiannually) is to get alignment of collaborators at each level, relative to how closely (or how far apart) they rate their own and others' performances, and to use the feedback process as a means of discussing ways of getting agreement on what each can do to achieve a more consensual alignment. In these two-way communication discussions or conferences, participants in the collaboration can gather information about those behaviors that need to be modified or changed in order to realize their goals or achieve their objectives. The alignment of the raters should show more consensus, as raters become more familiar with each other and the rating system, and should have a positive effect on the collaboration.

CONSIDERATIONS IN IMPLEMENTING MULTIRATER FEEDBACK PROCESS

Orientation/training sessions are essential for the raters, to reduce the amount of error. A few practice rounds of rating may be necessary, in order to build trust and confidence among raters in the process, so caution is urged in the interpretation of early ratings. To the extent possible, the process should ensure that the raters are anonymous, especially at the peer or colleague level. Raters should also have sufficient knowledge of the person(s) they are rating and should be informed about the working relationships of the person(s) they are rating. Additionally, the rating dimensions should focus specifically on job- or performance-related behaviors that are changeable, and not on personality or character traits. Because of the complexity involved in this type of process, it is probably wiser to begin with a pilot project, before full implementation is recommended for usage.

The two-way communication between the raters about feedback, with follow-up and follow-on, is important, because it increases the chances that the behavior changes are more likely to be perceived by those doing the ratings. It also increases the probability that the feedback will be used positively, because participants are more likely to ask for further clarification and feedback, if it is directly related to the suggestions they receive through multirater feedback. Specifically, this is because information from multiple raters produces a more complete picture of a person's behavior than does single-source feedback. Consequently, feedback reporting should be focused on cumulative scores, rather than on individual scores.

A major implication for using this kind of interactive assessment is that the promise for creating an environment in which participants in the collaboration can be empowered far surpasses a traditional approach to evaluation. Also, multirater feedback is likely to be more acceptable to the raters and more effective in assessing the process of the collaboration, if the dimensions have been developed with the participation of those who will be raters and those who will be rated. Through the multirater feedback process, the question, Did we do what we said we would do? is answered directly, leaving only the question, Did it matter?

Obviously, the proposed process requires support for the follow-up and follow-on of feedback recommendations, if it is to be successful. That is a major concern for the types of coalitions or collaborations that are the focus of this book, because of the need for infrastructure support for the introduction and implementation of a multirater feedback approach.

As mentioned, collaborations are virtual organizations, which do not have training and development programs and personnel in place to help the participants learn how to accept and give feedback and how to make the desired behavior changes. The budgets of participating organizations and individuals are not likely to have sufficient financial or human resources necessary for the development and support of a multirater feedback approach.

Multirater feedback processes require time and effort to develop the instruments, complete assessment forms, conduct feedback and clarification sessions, and develop action plans. These activities are costly, but critical, to the long-term success of a multirater feedback approach. Therefore, the funding agency must necessarily underwrite the developmental, administrative, support, and processing costs, as well as provide the technical assistance that will be necessary in the implementation stage of the process.

AN INCOMPLETE CASE STUDY

The question of whether a multirater approach can work in a public sector organization has only been partially answered. The author, while serving as a consultant, had some success in applying an adaptation of the model to a Los Angeles County shelter for children.

In July of 2000, the author was retained as a consultant, to facilitate a change from a traditional program service model to an integrated service model, for MacLaren Children's Center, a facility that provides temporary shelter services to wards of the court. The Los Angeles County Board of Supervisors had just enacted an ordinance to phase in staffing resources "to support and coordinate collaborative policy development initiatives, to assist County Departments to integrate service delivery systems, and to help provide children and families with needed information." The shelter has services provided by six separate departments, including an on-site school. Each department had a separate administrative structure, budget, system of reporting relationships, and salary scale. The author's task was to "assist managers, supervisors, and line staff with the transition to a fully integrated and results-based operating structure, which is able to measurably demonstrate improved outcomes for children and families."

Over the course of the next 13 months, the author conducted an assessment of the organization, conducted interviews with managers and supervisors, held focus group discussions with all levels of line staff, and held general orientations sessions on integrated service delivery systems. Weekly meetings were held with the administrator and management team, biweekly with the midlevel managers, and monthly with the supervisors, to facilitate and strengthen their collaborative efforts by building teams.

Six months into the process, the county introduced a strategic planning process with specified goals for management personnel, from which, over the next 4 months, the development of team goals was facilitated, with specific performance behaviors for each level, through supervision. The result was an accountability system in which all goals, objectives, and performance behaviors were tied to each other, regardless of departmental affiliation. A visible change occurred, with regularly scheduled staff meetings, sharing of information, and improved lines of reporting relationships.

The multirater approach was introduced to the management team, as a means of further developing the teams and as a means of evaluating the process of the collaboration. Over the next 2 months, we worked through an understanding of how the approach could work, and decided that we would first test it with senior managers and midlevel managers. The progress report was completed, as was a schedule for implementing the multirater system. However, before we could train the raters, personnel changes occurred, in which the administrator and several key managers were transferred to other county assignments, as the result of an internal audit on the care of children at the facility. A series of interim administrators were appointed, and the process was halted. Although we were unable to carry this process through to its conclusion, the limited amount of success convinced the author that the multirater approach can be designed and adapted as a useful tool in evaluating and developing collaborative efforts.

CONCLUSIONS

Today, institutions, organizations, and individuals in public and private sectors of our society are being asked to collaborate with each other, in order to solve some of the most pressing social and economic problems. These collaborations are taking many forms (coalitions, partnerships, etc.), most of which fall outside the norms of traditional organizational responses to social problems. Much of the impetus for this collective problem-solving approach has to do with the realization that few, if any, organizations have sufficient financial and human resources to address the myriad of problems we face.

On the other hand, pressure has come from governmental and private foundation funding guidelines, which encourage and even require interagency and interdisciplinary collaborations, public–private partnerships, community consultations, and citizen oversight. The objectives of such groupings are aimed at developing a more coordinated approach to providing human services. At organizational and community levels, this has taken the form of an integrated service approach, that is, several human services entities coming together, in carefully structured partnerships or joint ventures, to deliver services from a single point of accountability (Backer & Howard, 1999).

These initiatives have also created virtual organizations—collections of disciplines and individuals, which, although distinguished in their professional practices, do not have the infrastructure of personnel and resources to support and carry out the tasks that are critical to their success. Consequently, if they are to be successful, infrastructure support must be provided from elsewhere. A second issue of concern, which is addressed in this chapter, has to do with the problem of evaluating the effectiveness of these team-oriented collaborations. Subsequent to these givens is the demand for evaluative/assessment tools that not only meet the complexities of the virtual organizations created, but that also meet the demand of the dynamic, changing environment. Thus, the context of a complex, changing environment has been set, in which these collaborative efforts are to take place.

Further complicating these collaborative efforts are the realities that many of them are taking place in groups in which many cultures and subgroups are represented, bringing with them issues of ethnicity, culture, race, gender, class, and power. Our research and practice experience lead us to conclude that, unless these issues are addressed in a forthright manner, they are likely to inhibit the success of collaborative efforts, no matter how well-intended the actions of the collaborators might be. On the other hand, we found that there were several factors that could contribute to the success of these groupings whether they were assembled under the rubric of coalitions, collaborations, alliances, or partnerships. We referred to all of these collaborative efforts as partnerships, because that seemed to be the general nature of them all.

Major issues of mistrust of sponsoring institutions, or of the collaborative process itself, can present insurmountable barriers to the success of holding the partnership together, regardless of whether it met the original goals that were intended. Frequently, the success of these various partnerships depended upon their ability to empower disenfranchised groups and to deal positively with conflict that arose from the diversity of the coalitions themselves. Success, in these instances, focused as much on whether the coalition or collaboration stayed intact, as on how effective they were. It was obvious to us that, in order to determine the effectiveness of the collaborative efforts, as well as the virtual organization itself, more research was needed, and different approaches needed to be taken.

This chapter argues for the borrowing and adaptation of a multirater feedback approach to development/evaluation from private sector organizations that have made successful transitions from one organizational form to another, using the collaborative approach. The basis for a different approach to evaluation is the belief that traditional evaluation methodologies will not be successful when they are applied to nontraditional forms of organization, and that what is required is an evaluation strategy that is aligned with the team-oriented approach that collaboration represents.

The multirater feedback approach is offered as both a developmental and evaluative tool that is not only consistent with the integrated service approach, but one that involves the participants in the collaboration in an active role of assessing their performances through self–other appraisals. The application of this model creates new roles for all involved, including the funding agencies, by developing an interactive accountability system, based on specific performance behaviors that are linked to shared goals and objectives. In the human services, we are apparently faced with a transformational moment: The unsettled question is, Will we take advantage of it?

REFERENCES

Abramson, J., & Rosenthal, B. (1995). Interdisciplinary and interorganizational collaboration. In R. Edwards (Ed.), *The encyclopedia of social work* (19th ed., pp. 1479–1489). Washington, DC: National Association of Social Workers.

Backer, T. E., & Howard, E. A. (1999). *Integrated service programs for women with multiple vulnerabilities.* Culver City, CA: PROTOTYPES Systems Change Center.

Backer, T. E., & Norman, A. J. (1998). *Best practices in multicultural coalitions: Phase I report to the California Endowment.* Northridge, CA: Human Interaction Research Institute.

Backer, T. E., & Norman, A. J. (2000, September). Partnerships and community change. *California Politics and Policy, 39–44.*

Bernadin, H. J., & Beatty, R. W. (1987, Summer). Can subordinate appraisals enhance managerial productivity? *Sloan Management Review, 63–73.*

Harris, M. M., & Schaubroeck, J. (1988). A meta-analysis of self-supervisor, self-peer, and peer-supervisor ratings. *Personnel Psychology, 41, 43–59.*

Latham, G. P., & Wexley, K. N. (1982). *Increasing productivity through performance appraisal.* Reading, MA: Addison-Wesley.

Lewis, J. A. (2001). The domains of human service organizations. In J. A. Lewis (Ed.), M. D. Lewis, & F. Souflee, Jr., *Management of human service programs* (pp. 1–11). Belmont, CA: Wadsworth.

Lorsch, N. E., & Goodearle, H. (1994). *Multirater feedback: Human Resources Special Report.* Los Angeles: Hughes.

Norman, A. J. (1996). Building coalitions across ethnic/racial lines: Some practical issues for consideration. *California Politics and Policy, 71–73.*

Nowack, K. M. (1992). Self-assessment and rater-assessment as a dimension of management development. *Human Resource Quarterly, 3*(2), 141–157.

Nowack, K. M. (1993). 360-feedback: The whole story. *Training and Development, 69–72.*

Tornow, W. W. (1993). Editor's note: Introduction to special issue on 360-feedback. *Human Resource Management, 32*(2–3) 211–219.

CHAPTER 3

The Human Side of
Evaluating Collaborations

Thomas E. Backer and Cynthia D. Kunz

- A community-wide collaboration reports, confidentially, that it is experiencing massive "collaboration fatigue." There are so many partnerships going on in its community, with key leaders sitting on not one, but a number of them, that people are simply getting tired of collaborating. But no one will say this for the record or in public, because they fear negative reactions from funders who want them to be involved in these collaborations.
- Everything about the work of a community collaboration on youth violence prevention is changed by the devastating impact of a major flood that submerged large sections of the community's metropolitan area. Even 4 years later, the psychological and fiscal responses to community action are measured in terms of the urgency of simply recovering from the flood.
- A whole group of communities—recipients of youth violence prevention planning grants by a foundation—repeatedly express their consternation about the funder's determination, as a matter of policy, not to award implementation grants to the same nonprofit organization that received the planning grant. The funder is equally perplexed that, despite repeated communications about their policy, community collaboration leaders continue to plan for a transition from the planning to

implementation grant within the organization. The resulting tension affects what otherwise is a rather positive funder–community relationship.

- A youth violence prevention collaboration wrestles with the difficulty of getting direct involvement of youth in their activities. Any outside observer can easily see that one of the problems is their reluctance to share power with young people, even though their objectives are directed at youth development services.
- A case study of a grant project in which a collaboration played a key role, prepared by an independent evaluator and based on review of grantee reports and interviews, provokes serious negative reactions from the grantee. The rewritten case report seems to provide a more accurate picture of the project as it had actually unfolded, but is at serious variance with what was said by the grantee in its original project reports.
- The director of a grant project that had ended before the evaluation took place resists participating in the evaluative process. As a result, no interview material is available, and there is no one inside the project to review a case study report prepared about it that is based on previously submitted grantee reports.
- A grant project with a collaboration element provides very thin and not particularly informative reports on the project. It does not receive second-year funding, which causes outside evaluators to initially suspect that the consensus-building process has not been successful. Telephone interviews, however, reveal that this was, in fact, a successful project and that second-year funding had been turned down because sufficient local resources were in place and the grantee did not wish to deal with further funder bureaucracy, especially "silly paperwork."
- A collaboration-based project desires to replicate a successful innovation for providing services to individuals in rural areas. A major roadblock surfaces, however: the unwillingness of service personnel to deliver the services directly in these rural areas. The initial stated reason is diversion of time from other work (including travel time), but what later emerges is that these people often feel unsafe in very remote areas, especially when dealing with clients with a history of violence, or whose propensity toward violence is unknown.

These brief case examples present just a sampling of the human complexities that can affect the operation and success of collaborations and their evaluation. Some reflect individual fears, resistances, and concerns about the collaboration or about the evaluation process. Others are the positive feelings (and outcomes) that emerge when people learn to work well together in a collaboration, to find new ways to trust and communicate with one another across cultural and value divides, to allow leadership to supercede turf issues, to build consensus, even when there is not unanimous agreement. Sometimes, the fears and resistances, in fact, are overcome by the collaboration members' willingness to set them aside in order to reach a desired goal of systems change (including making use of suggestions that emerge from an evaluation).

Still others are a function of group dynamics, which are also a powerful source of either positive or negative drive for the kind of systems change (in an organization's or community's program, procedure, or policy) to which most collaborations are directed. The group involved may be the collaboration or it may be the entire community in which the collaboration exists. At both the individual and group levels, this human side of change may stem from specific reactions to particular events or goals of a collaboration, or it may reflect underlying culture or history within the community.

Evaluators must be sensitive to these human complexities, because they affect both process and outcomes of a collaboration. And, in the case of individual or group reactions to the evaluation process itself, the evaluators' actions may themselves help to shape outcomes in either helpful or troublesome ways. Evaluation is by its nature an emotion-laden topic for nonprofit and community leaders involved with a collaboration. The emotions can range from excitement about the chance to improve a collaboration's effectiveness, to fear about possible adverse consequences from an evaluator's report, to anger that a community effort is being subjected to outside scrutiny because of a funder's demand.

A collaboration is inherently a human enterprise. It has no life but the complex human life of the people who make it up. This is true, even though most people participating in a collaboration are there representing an organization, a group, or a community. Evaluations that focus only on the procedures or the outcomes of a collaboration, and do not look at the living people who make it up or at their personal reactions to the collaboration process, are not likely to yield the most accurate or helpful portrait of the collaboration's work and success.

Although not even close to an exhaustive list of human reactions to collaboration evaluation, the examples above reflect the following challenges:

- Collaboration fatigue
- Emotions resulting from larger events in the community
- Reactions to funder's rules about collaborations they support

- Reluctance to share power and authority
- Negative reactions to an outside evaluator's report
- Resistance to participating in the evaluation process
- Resistance to the overall bureaucracy required by a funder
- Personal concerns about participation in certain aspects of a collaboration

The eight examples just given all come from two recent evaluations the authors' organization carried out, one for the John S. and James L. Knight Foundation's "Initiative to Prevent Youth Violence and Promote Youth Development" (Backer, 2001) and another for the federal Center for Mental Health Services' (CMHS's) Community Action Grant program (Backer, Howard, & Koone, 2000). Both were evaluations of a group of projects in which collaborations played a central role, and both required special sensitivity to the human issues these complex situations raise.

What follows is an exploration of how these human dynamics are identified and analyzed and what to do about them when problems occur as part of a collaboration's evaluation. This discussion focuses on the works of external evaluations commissioned to do their work by a collaboration funder, but much of what is said here also would apply to an internal evaluation conducted by, or at least commissioned by, the collaboration itself.

WHERE HUMAN PROBLEMS OCCUR

As the previous examples make clear, problems emerging from the complex individual and group dynamics of the many actors in a collaboration can occur at many levels, including:

- *Definition.* People involved in a collaboration frequently differ in their understanding of what the collaboration actually is as a community body.
- *Goals.* People in a collaboration often differ on what they see as the near-term and ultimate goals the collaboration is supposed to accomplish.
- *Involvement.* Who should be at the table often is a sensitive issue, especially in diverse communities, where even accidental exclusion of a certain group can provoke hard feelings and real difficulties for the collaboration's success.

- *Operation.* Who sets the operating strategy for the collaboration, in effect, determining "who does what to whom" in its everyday operations.
- *Process.* How the collaboration functions in handling conflicts, making decisions, and sustaining itself over time.
- *Outcomes.* What constitutes a measure of success for a collaboration also can be a source of disagreement.
- *Evaluation.* How to actually do that measuring, including the time costs of evaluation, the possibility of incomplete or mistaken interpretations, and who gets to settle any disputes over the meaning of evaluation results.

All of these are human issues, because they involve perception and judgment, and also involve differing values and aspirations. One of the reasons is that collaborations are inherently human enterprises, which depend on goodwill, mutual understanding, and trust. They are voluntary enterprises, and are often nonfunded, so it is the motivation of the participants that drives them. For this reason alone, collaborations have a low chance of survival if the human issues surrounding them are not attended to reasonably well. This is true at each stage in the life cycle: development, implementation, and long-term maintenance.

Emphasizing the human issues, as is done here, may obscure the fact that seldom are participants free agents. Rather, they are representatives of organizations and, as such, have a whole set of other dynamics with which they must deal. Thus, there may be enormous differences in dealing with a neighborhood committee (all independent actors) and a collaboration (all representing institutions and not themselves).

EVALUATION APPROACHES THAT EMPHASIZE THE HUMAN ELEMENT

Evaluators need to be sensitive to these issues and to their own participation in, and impact on, the collaboration process. In most of the approaches used today, evaluators are not totally objective and are part of the ongoing stream of events.

Evaluation theory and practice help with this. Four pertinent approaches are:

- *Empowerment evaluation* (Fetterman, Kaftarian, & Wandersman, 1996) concentrates on involving stakeholders in each stage of designing, carrying out, and reporting results from an evaluation.

- *Developmental evaluation* (Patton, 1994) is a more concentrated effort, along the lines of process evaluation, to weave together the evaluation process as part of the long-term natural development of a community program.
- *Utilization-focused evaluation* (Patton, 1986) is focused on how to conduct evaluations so that their results can be used to improve the program, change policy, or otherwise positively affect the life of the community.
- A *clinical approach to evaluation* (Glaser & Backer, 1972) rests on the assumption that assessments will be most meaningful and useful if they are designed to evaluate the program as a whole and as a dynamic, complexly interrelated entity, with careful attention to the thoughts, feelings, and beliefs of all those who are concerned with a program.

Each of these approaches are referred to later, as ways of dealing with the issues raised here. What all share is a philosophy: Meaningful and accurate evaluation requires ongoing communication with, and involvement of, those whose work is being evaluated or who are affected by the collaboration. For the purposes of this chapter, that includes funders, policy makers and other community leaders, and, of course, the target populations who may benefit from whatever the collaboration achieves.

THE LARGER CONTEXT OF CHANGE

As stated, collaborations are formed to create systems change in some community system—to design a new program, implement a procedure, or change a policy that will improve services or quality of life in that community. The system involved may be a single organization, a whole group of them working together, or the community as a whole. When evaluating a collaboration's process or outcomes, it is essential to put that specific systems change, and the work of the collaboration, into the larger context of three principles about change (which have been culled from more than 100 years of management and behavioral science; see Backer, 1997, 2000):

- *Systems change happens only when individual people change.*
- *The complex psychological responses people and groups have to change must be addressed, or failure is likely.*
- *The nature of change itself is changing at multiple levels.*

Systems Change Happens Only When Individual People Change

In their 1996 book, *Paradox Principles*, the Price Waterhouse Change Integration Team says it elegantly: "Personal change is the prerequisite to organizational change. . . . Organizational transformation occurs one individual at a time" (p. 2). Yet, far too many systems change efforts become diverted with fancy theoretical models, organizational diagrams, flow charts, and other ways of looking at the system, without focusing on the individuals in it. This is dangerous.

The Complex Psychological Responses People and Groups Have to Change Must Be Addressed, or Failure Is Likely

Every organization is a living museum of its past change efforts, many of which fail to work, or, at least, work well. Sometimes financial, political, or other realities create failure. Unplanned change can overtake planned change: A party loses power in Congress, an earthquake happens, a budget gets slashed. Sometimes, the change program itself is inherently flawed. But, more often, change efforts fail because there is insufficient creative and strategic attention to how people respond psychologically when asked to make significant changes at work. Ironically, this often occurs despite intellectual understanding that change is hard. And it occurs despite a sincere conviction that paying attention to human responses to change is important. The failure is at the implementation level: lack of foresight and planning, and poorly executed interventions to help people at the firing-line level—staff, clients, and families—deal with two fundamental aspects of change:

- Their resistances, fears, and anxieties about change, or even the contemplation of it
- Their needs to participate in planning for change, and to feel individually rewarded for their involvement in the change, not just abstractly, but in ways that are directly relevant to their work and lives

Strategies for handling these aspects are well-documented in the behavioral sciences literature, but are often neglected in planning for systems change and the long-term health of the collaboration that is helping to promote that change. Change efforts in health and social services are especially likely to downplay these human dimensions, because service professionals think they already know how to "do change." After all, change through therapeutic intervention is our business, and we think our commitment to a service goal makes us somehow immune to the dynamics of change we would always address if we were advising a client, a family, or a private business about change.

The most dangerous situations, in fact, are those in which everybody agrees the change is desirable, there are resources to make it happen, and no enemies of change are around. But resistance to change is still almost inevitable, and, even if not expressed openly, the "subtle sabotage of withheld enthusiasm" may scuttle the transformation, or at least significantly compromise it. In the former Soviet Union, people were sent to the Gulag or even executed for resisting change, and still they resisted. Writing in *Fortune* magazine, Anne Fisher (1995) says "Change is painful. Pushed to change the way they work, most people push back. Every change, no matter how innocuous or even beneficial it may seem on the surface, costs somebody something" (p. 121).

The corporate world also reflects this reality. In a 1995 *Harvard Business Review* article called "Why Transformation Efforts Fail," Harvard Business School professor John Kotter reports the results of his decade-long study of more than 100 companies. Kotter studied programs involving total quality management, reengineering, rightsizing, restructuring, organization-wide cultural change, and corporate turnarounds. His results are discouraging: "A few of these corporate change efforts have been very successful. A few have been utter failures. Most fall somewhere in between, with a distinct tilt toward the lower end of the scale" (p. 62).

MIT's Michael Hammer, the leading guru of reengineering, says that two thirds of reengineering interventions have failed, mostly because of staff resistance. Human beings' innate resistance to change is "the most perplexing, annoying, distressing, and confusing part" of reengineering, says Hammer. Resistance to change

> is natural and inevitable. To think that resistance won't occur or to view those who exhibit its symptoms as difficult or retrograde is a fatal mistake. . . . The real cause of reengineering failures is not the resistance itself but management's failure to deal with it. (p. 114)

Evaluators of collaborations are more likely to reveal how and why a collaboration has worked—or has not—if they pay sensitive attention to these complex human reactions. As stated earlier, not all human responses to change are negative, however. There is also a positive side to the involvement of people and groups in collaborations, which need to be measured by evaluators, in order to understand both what has happened in a collaboration and why it has been successful. People learn to work well together and to find new ways to communicate with each other across cultural and value divides. Leadership sometimes supercedes turf issues, and consensus is achieved even when there is not unanimous agreement. Evaluators' suggestions are acted upon even when they create discomfort, because they are seen as contributing to the improvement of the collaboration's work and ultimate impact. People and groups derive a sense of satisfaction and accomplishment from the work of change (e.g., "Finally, our community is making a difference on this issue!").

The Nature of Change Itself Is Changing at Multiple Levels

The first level is *complexity*. Given the challenges nonprofit organizations and communities are facing today, there are simply more kinds of systems change efforts going on at the local level, and at the state, national, and world levels as well. This probably includes the work of other collaborations within a given community. Evaluators may not have the resources to examine these other systems change efforts or determine their impact on the collaboration they are studying, but simply recognizing that this larger complexity of systems change exists can change the interpretive frame of an evaluation. For instance, if a collaboration's work in a community is resisted, might part of the reason be that there is so much other change happening at a particular point in time that people and groups in the community are too exhausted to take on another effort, no matter how worthy they may feel it to be?

Also, evaluators can usefully explore whether a collaboration's leadership takes account of the larger context for their work. Are they perhaps losing credibility because they act as if "our change is the only change going on," or are they actively looking for opportunities to achieve synergy with other change efforts, and to avoid possible timing errors related to when they introduce certain aspects of their own systems change work, against the backdrop of all the other change happening in a community?

The second level is *pace*. In today's environment, the pace of change is increasing in every area of activity. Collaborations are affected by this increasing pace, because it tightens up their own time frames for success; those that do not respond may get left in the dust by other ongoing change in their own communities. Evaluators can better understand the impact of a collaboration by looking at how these responses are made or not made.

The third level is *diminishing resources and destabilization*. The work of collaborations addressing everything from human services to the arts has been profoundly affected by the recent economic downturn in America and by the tragic events of September 11, for example. If it was not already true, these enormous events have implemented fully what Tom Peters (1987) wrote about in *Thriving on Chaos* almost 15 years ago: There is a paradigm shift going on in the world, not just to a new set of rules, but to a world in which the rules keep changing. Economic futurist Hazel Henderson puts it another way, saying that the fundamental logic error of our time is "assuming that anything will ever go back to the way it was" (Backer, 1997, p. 445).

Again, evaluators of collaborations must look at how individuals and groups within a collaboration are reacting to these realities. Are they hiding behind old, outdated assumptions, or are they frozen into inaction? Or are they using this time of diminished resources and destabilization as an opportunity to re-sort priorities, unstick resistance, and move ahead, even if the movement is to an altered goal, given the new realities? Is there more resistance to evaluation than before, because of these new threats and the uncertainty they introduce? Or is there a greater desire for evaluation that may help to identify strategies that can be effective in this dramatically changed environment?

THE TROUBLED COLLABORATION

Some collaborations run fairly smoothly during their development and operation; others are fraught with dysfunction, including poorly managed conflict among the collaboration participants (or between the collaboration and some element of the larger community). Conflict over basic values or operating strategies may be quite healthy, if participants in the collaboration have set procedures for handling such disagreements, or bring in an outside mediator to help resolve the issues. But at other times it is a warning sign of what may be more profound troubles of deep cultural divides, financial or legal problems, or other unforeseen circumstances.

Outside evaluators may have two different roles in relation to such elements of the troubled collaboration. Dysfunctions, or even crises, of the collaboration are legitimate material for the evaluation. In some cases, understanding them may be central to learning why a collaboration has not succeeded well in its stated mission, or to suggesting, through the evaluation process, steps that might be taken to improve the collaboration's function. Evaluators also need to be sensitive to troubles in the collaboration's operation, because sometimes they can lead to seriously distorted evaluation findings, for example, when a collaboration's members may feel ashamed or threatened by the disclosure of their troubles and try to conceal them. In most instances, although there may be no drive to concealment, collaboration participants will be distracted from the time and energy they might otherwise contribute to the evaluation process, making it impossible to obtain needed evaluation data or access to collaboration members or staff.

A second and more delicate role occurs when an evaluator becomes aware that a collaboration is troubled and either is asked by collaboration members (or funders, community leaders outside the collaboration, etc.) to intervene, or independently decides that some intervention by the evaluator might be possible. This may involve sharing evaluation findings that can be used by others to formulate an intervention, with the possibility of negative reactions from some who do not want "dirty laundry" aired.

If it is almost any other type of intervention, evaluators must proceed very carefully, to maintain their objectivity and credibility with other actors on the scene. Even if the collaboration is a new, volunteer-driven enterprise that has little structure for dealing with its own difficulties, the evaluator's typical role does not make intervention of any sort easy, and there may be straightforward ethical issues, too, about getting involved. On the other hand, an evaluator with a well-established, positive relationship with collaboration members of staff may be able to intervene discreetly and helpfully, in part because they have an outsider's objectivity. Sometimes, the evaluator's objectivity in reframing contentious issues may be exactly what the collaboration needs to resolve a conflict and move ahead.

In many cases, evaluators of a collaboration may find it desirable to set up, in advance, structures by which they will or will not become involved in any sort of intervention when trouble is detected. This may require agreement not only by the collaboration members, but also by the funder of the collaboration and the evaluation, and possibly by other stakeholders as well.

How will evaluators be likely to determine that a collaboration is troubled? Because community collaborations, by their very nature, require that people come together as individuals and as representatives of community interests and organizations, evaluators should be sensitive to the nature and quality of the group's behavior. Evaluators may receive overt signals that the group is in trouble, such as failure to meet joint goals over time, or active complaints from participants. In these cases, and provided that the terms of the evaluator's engagement allow, the suggestion that third-party or neutral assistance from a facilitator or mediator be considered is probably an appropriate one to make (see Fisher & Ury, 1991; *Harvard Business Review*, 2000; and Ury, 1993 for basic information about mediation and conflict resolution).

Evaluators should, however, be sensitive to the presence of more subtle signs that a group may be in trouble or may be developing the kinds of trouble that mean their common purpose will be compromised. Some of the signs that facilitators and mediators see, when troubled community collaborations convene and conduct their meetings, include the following:

Before the meeting:

- Lack of regularity, in schedules, agendas, or meeting reports
- Lack of order, such as uncertain start times, or late arrivals

During the meeting:

- Lack of meeting focus
- Sidebar, dyadic, or triadic discussions, while meeting is going on
- Individuals disassociating from the group, leaving early
- Lack of compromise in discussions
- Sarcasm in verbal communications
- Lack of humor, spontaneity, enthusiasm
- Lack of reinforcement of opinion, appreciative inquiry, or affirming behavior
- Vague allusions to past problems

Discoveries over time:

- Excessive turnover in membership representation
- Absenteeism among representatives
- Failure to meet expected outcomes
- Withholding of necessary data or communications
- Dissonance in terminology describing purposes and function

None of these signs, of themselves, necessarily spells failure in the group's process or purposes. Representatives sometimes simply have bad days; external events may have a negative effect on the ability of the group to function; and even healthy groups do sometimes seem to test their own limits. The presence of more than a few of these signs, more than a few times, does, however, strongly suggest the presence of issues and problems capable of compromising a group's common purpose—issues and problems that the evaluator may not be in a position to address.

Sometimes, in fact, the trouble may be between the evaluator and the collaboration itself. Outside evaluations may create resentments or feelings of intrusion or defensiveness from collaboration members or other community leaders, and these may be accentuated if the evaluators come from a culture different from that of many in the collaboration. Even for internally conducted evaluations, there may be negative feelings about the use of scarce resources to do the evaluation, instead of doing the direct work of the collaboration. In these cases, evaluators need to do all they can to hang on to their objectivity, to ask for feedback that may be useful either in reshaping the evaluation or in providing more input to the collaboration members or community about why it needs to be carried out in a certain way.

EVALUATOR INTERVENTIONS

What we have found in studying collaborations and coalitions is that evaluation designs, data-gathering and analysis strategies, reporting methods, and especially communications between the evaluator and the collaboration, can all be shaped to address the challenges just mentioned. For instance, if there is an ongoing problem or conflict in the collaboration, an evaluator may be able to refer collaborative leadership to a professional who specializes in conflict analysis, management, and resolution, who can help to lessen or resolve the conflict.

As mentioned, the first step is simply for evaluators to be sensitive to these human and institutional dimensions. Program evaluators are often trained and acculturated in a tradition of the social or behavioral sciences that prizes objectivity and looks for clean measures that do not involve subjective reactions or opinions. Although objective measures may have great value, they miss capturing the more emotional, subjective elements that often determine outcomes in significant ways, and this is particularly true with something as relatively new on the scene as a collaboration.

Evaluators are often in a unique position to identify and begin to address conflict, as well as a host of related dysfunctions, experienced by collaboration groups. Depending upon the terms of their engagement, evaluators can have relatively open access to collaboration participants and to their activities, interactions, thoughts, beliefs, and judgments. Because of the general importance attached to any evaluation effort in publicly funded human service endeavors, evaluators can also come to enjoy a unique position of trust among both collaboration leaders and participants. Again, depending upon the terms of engagement, some evaluators can play a quasi-consultant role, in which early findings from utilization-focused or developmental evaluations are used to highlight the appearance of problems, performance deficits, and emergent or active conflict.

When evaluation results suggest the presence of any of these, evaluators can themselves turn, or can suggest a referral, to institutional mediators and others with professional preparation in conflict analysis, management, and resolution. Unlike evaluators, these specialists are trained to help groups grapple with a range of real and perceived issues that generally characterize a troubled collaboration. In general, they will wear a different set of lenses when working with a collaboration and its participants, viewing individuals, certainly, but objectifying the parties and their separate interests and focusing on the structure and processes with which they work together.

In some cases, a mediator's intervention is as straightforward as revisiting with a collaborating group the several necessary steps and issues associated with solid group performance and discussing what can, and often does, go wrong. A faltering collaboration may find, for example, that it has acquired new members or representatives over time, but has neglected to pause to orient, establish trust, clarify roles, and secure commitment from them.

In other cases, specific collaboration decisions (or indecisions) have generated controversy or active conflict, for which the group as a whole was unprepared or with which it was unable to respond productively. A mediator's intervention can help collaborations address existing conflict and often resolve it, in whole or in part, by negotiating resolution strategies among the parties. A mediator's intervention can also help collaborations better prepare themselves for the real potential for difference and disagreement, in order to prevent active conflict before it emerges and to better manage it when it does.

In still other cases, a mediator's intervention can help a struggling collaboration come to grips with difficult kinds of realities. For example, there comes a time for some groups when they have accomplished what was intended and either need to disband and move on or explore a renewed purpose. There may come a time for other groups when they realize their purpose is unachievable without substantial restructuring or the addition of new members and representatives. There may also come a time when external events or pressures (e.g., budget cuts and changes in funding priority) force collaborations to consider more formalized mechanisms of working together, including functional and other mergers designed to reduce costs.

Unfortunately, for some groups, not all troubles are resolvable among the parties in the classic sense. Where there has been wrongdoing of some kind (for example, malfeasance, discrimination, or violation of other rights and standards), a mediator's intervention can help sort out matters and, with appropriate legal support, help to manage the consequences and the aftermath.

Because evaluators often see early signs and signals of trouble, but are not necessarily prepared either professionally or by the terms of engagement to address these in meaningful ways, the assistance of, or referral to, conflict resolution specialists can be very helpful. Preventing conflict is generally easier and much less costly in both financial and human terms than managing or resolving it. Evaluators are often the first neutral or third party on the scene and can play a unique role in assuring that these signs and signals are heard and correctly interpreted, before the trouble they herald overcomes a collaboration's ability to meet its goals.

Human and institutional and group dimensions also can be positively addressed by involving the collaboration's membership more actively in designing and carrying out the evaluation (Glaser & Backer, 1972). This will not solve other problems in the organization, but it may increase positive support for the evaluation and may open channels of communication, which can improve both its feasibility and quality. Empowerment approaches to evaluation (discussed in the Foreword to this book and elsewhere in the volume) are certainly worth considering, because of this potential benefit.

Utilization-focused evaluation (Patton, 1986) can be of significant value, because it focuses appropriate attention on what will be done with the results of evaluation—how findings can be used to improve a program, change public policy, and instigate other kinds of change in the community where the evaluation took place. And developmental evaluation (Patton, 1994) can help to more successfully shape the implementation of a collaboration (and the work it is addressing), by tying together evaluators and collaboration personnel in the conjoint effort of using evaluation data to improve the program itself.

The clinical approach to evaluation (Glaser & Backer, 1972) suggests five specific activities, in addition to more traditional evaluation measurement approaches, such as survey questionnaires, each of which may be helpful to consider in dealing with complex human and institutional and group dynamics:

1. *Subjective measurement.* Methods for obtaining the opinions or judgments of people in a program (staff and service recipients).
2. *Consultation.* Using a consultation model (which assumes peer status, rather than an authority relationship) to direct interaction between collaboration members and the evaluators.
3. *Feedback.* Providing information immediately, whenever it might be useful for program improvement (again, as in the developmental approach), rather than waiting until the end of the evaluation.
4. *Debriefing.* Interacting with collaboration staff about the evaluation results, beginning with sharing of draft reports that can be reviewed

editorially by the collaboration members or staff, so that additions or corrections to errors of fact can be made as needed.

5. *Participant observation.* Actually bringing evaluation staff into the routine activities of the collaboration (sitting in on meetings, for instance), so that there is a chance to grasp the living process of the collaboration.

The Knight evaluation (Backer, 2001) mentioned earlier began with an *evaluability assessment* (an established methodology in the program evaluation field), which involved a preliminary scan of each of the planning grants in their environments (through interviews and document review), then development of the design for a full evaluation. During this early assessment phase, concern by members of the collaborations about the transition from planning to implementation grant in their communities came to light, as did the common occurrence of spin-off projects that were enabled by the planning grants, but not formal outcomes. The evaluation design was shaped to capture information about both elements, and the opportunity to influence that design appeared to increase openness of the collaboration members in talking about their experiences.

A main evaluation tool for both the evaluability assessment and the full planning grant evaluation was a narrative-form case study report based upon interviews and document analysis. Prior to being submitted to the funder, these case studies were reviewed in draft form by the collaboration members interviewed. This also helped to develop trust and openness regarding the evaluation process, as well as increasing accuracy and completeness.

The same procedure was used as a major element of the CMHS Community Action Grant evaluation, with the same result (Backer, Howard, and Koone, 2000). Even when there were negative reactions to the content of the draft report (which happened in only 1 of 17 cases), the collaboration members involved were willing to review the draft document and explain how they thought it could be fixed to make it more accurate (and most of these suggestions were in fact implemented).

Both evaluations included an informal search, through patient interactions with interviewees, for unanticipated outcomes. The planning grant spin-off projects, identified for the Youth Violence Prevention Initiative evaluation, were a major find. These were cited later by the foundation's leadership, in a memorandum to the Knight board of trustees, as one of the great benefits of this planning grants program.

The CMHS Community Action Grant evaluation also included a content analysis of written reports submitted by the grantees, including a focus on the collaboration process itself: issues raised in collaboration meetings and how these were addressed by each project; how stakeholder readiness among the collaboration members was assessed and what changes were made in the operation of the project as a result; to what extent collaboration members bought into the innovative program the collaboration was attempting to implement; and how consensus was achieved by the collaboration members to implement the innovation.

These approaches to evaluation may take some additional time to plan and implement, but the extra effort they require usually pays off, because of their sensitivity to the complex human issues that always are part of the larger context for evaluation. This is particularly true when evaluating collaborations, which, by their nature, involve diverse, often conflicting personalities and interests in the community.

CONCLUSIONS

Evaluators of collaborations (and indeed evaluators of any type of community intervention or program) are most likely to succeed in understanding process and assessing outcomes, if they begin with:

- sensitivity to the complex human and institutional and group elements driving the collaborations they are evaluating;
- a willingness to use appropriately some evaluation approaches that have been devised, in part, to address such concerns by collaboration members;
- a willingness to communicate with collaboration members on an ongoing basis, as a part of the natural process of the evaluation;
- a readiness to share findings (including drafts on which collaboration members can comment, leading to revisions, if necessary) from the evaluation, both to build trust and to help improve the collaboration; and
- a willingness to get involved more directly in crisis situations (with all the cautions previously stated), for example, by connecting a collaboration with a mediation expert, if there is conflict among the collaboration's leadership that needs to be resolved. There are a number of approaches in the evaluation literature, four of which are briefly described earlier, which can help to organize such responses.

Evaluators also need to measure and deal with their own human responses to the evaluation process—frustration that collaboration members are difficult to reach or are seemingly not forthcoming, or conflicting expectations from funders, for example. These can influence the interpretation of results significantly, if they are not handled in an appropriate way.

Moreover, evaluators need to regard their evaluative intervention as just one element in a more complex environment, in which other change efforts, other service programs, and other evaluations all coexist with each other and with the wild complexities of the world at large. Evaluation must be sensitive to this larger context of multicultural populations, the special features of specific content areas, such as youth violence prevention or mental health services for people with serious mental illness, the whole community, and even the framework. As discussed in the other chapters of this volume, there are specific materials and wisdom that relate to each one of these topics, to aid the evaluator of collaborations in this challenging task.

ACKNOWLEDGMENT

The authors acknowledge the helpful editorial input of Elizabeth Howard, Human Interaction Research Institute, to the development of this chapter.

REFERENCES

Backer, T. E. (1997). Managing the human side of change in VA's transformation. *Hospital and Health Services Administration, 42*(3), 433–439.

Backer, T. E. (2000). The failure of success: Challenges of disseminating effective substance abuse prevention programs. *Journal of Community Psychology, 28*(3), 363–373.

Backer, T. E. (2001). *Cross-site evaluation for the planning phase of Knight Foundation's Initiative to Promote Youth Development and Prevent Youth Violence.* Encino, CA: Human Interaction Research Institute.

Backer, T. E., Howard, E. A., & Koone, U. S. (2000). *Final report: Evaluation of the Community Action Grant program—Phase 1: Round 1 grantees.* Encino, CA: Human Interaction Research Institute.

Fetterman, R. M., Kaftarian, S. J., & Wandersman, A. (Eds.). (1996). *Empowerment evaluation: Knowledge and tools for self-assessment and accountability.* Thousand Oaks, CA: Sage.

Fisher, A. B. (1995, April 17). Making change stick. *Fortune,* 121–130.

Fisher, R., & Ury, W. (1991) *Getting to yes: Negotiating agreement without giving in.* New York: Penguin.

Glaser, E. M., & Backer, T. E. (1972). A clinical approach to program evaluation. *Evaluation, 1,* 54–59.

Hammer, M. (1995). *The re-engineering revolution.* Cambridge, MA: Massachusetts Institute of Technology.

Harvard Business Review. (2000) *Negotiation and conflict resolution.* Boston: Harvard Business School Publishing.

Kotter, J. P. (1995, March–April). Leading change: Why transformation efforts fail. *Harvard Business Review,* 59–67.

Moore, C. (1996). *The mediation process: Practical strategies for resolving conflict.* San Francisco: Jossey-Bass.

Patton, M. Q. (1986). *Utilization-focused evaluation.* Beverly Hills, CA: Sage.

Patton, M. Q. (1994). Developmental evaluation. *Evaluation Practice, 15,* 311–319.

Peters, T. (1987). *Thriving on chaos: Handbook for a management revolution.* New York: Harper Collins.

Price Waterhouse Change Integration Team. (1996). *Paradox principles.* Chicago: Irwin.

Ury, W. (1993). *Getting past no: Negotiating your way from confrontation to cooperation.* New York: Bantam.

CHAPTER 4

A Practical Approach to Evaluation of Collaborations

Tom Wolff

Those who work closely with collaborations on a regular basis know that the effectiveness varies widely in operations and outcomes from interventions labeled coalitions, collaborations, or partnerships. Some of this may result from the limitations on these interventions, even when performed at the highest level of effectiveness, to create all the community changes that the participants and funders may want. More often, ineffectiveness can be attributed to the poor design or implementation of the collaboration process. Thus, we not only must take a serious look at creating evaluations of collaboration outcomes, but also at creating mechanisms for collaborations to assess the effectiveness of their processes.

The minimal level of engagement of collaborations in effective evaluation processes can be attributed to at least three factors: (1) the motivation, interest, and intent of the collaboration to actually carry out an evaluation; (2) the failure of the collaboration to find appropriate evaluators and set up mutually effective and respectful relationships with them; and (3) the lack of access to easy, usable tools for evaluating the process and outcome of their collaboration efforts. This chapter addresses these issues by first discussing the process of engaging in an evaluation and the development of effective relationships with evaluators, then by illustrating examples of effective process and outcome tools, many of which can be used without the assistance of an outside evaluator.

WHY DO COLLABORATIONS BECOME ENGAGED IN EVALUATION?

For most collaborations, the motivation to engage in an evaluation process is that it is a requirement for their funding. Someone else has decided for them that evaluation is a necessity. Yet, successful evaluations most often occur when the collaboration itself decides that there are critical questions that must be answered, such as, After having been at this for three years, are we getting anything done? Are we being effective? Is the way that we are set up the most effective? and What do all of our members think about what we are doing? These kinds of questions can motivate a steering committee and staff of a collaboration to come into an evaluation process with a high level of interest and motivation.

HOW DO YOU BUILD OWNERSHIP IN COLLABORATIONS FOR THE EVALUATION PROCESS?

Collaboration evaluation is often a mystery for staff and members. As a result, collaborations often hire outside evaluators and leave the evaluation to them. They accept whatever recommendations are made, because the evaluators are the "experts." This is not necessary, nor is it recommended. The collaboration is the primary consumer of the evaluation, so the collaboration needs to be heavily engaged and invested in the evaluation process. Just as empowerment is an underlying principle for collaboration activities and functioning, empowerment must also be an underlying principle of the evaluation process.

Indeed, the concepts of empowerment evaluation (Fetterman, 1994) and participatory evaluation are increasingly popular approaches to the evaluation process. Participatory evaluation is a method in the family of action research that seeks to be practical, useful, informative, and empowering. Participatory evaluation approaches are practical, in that they respond to the needs, interests, and concerns of the collaboration; they are useful, because the findings are employed and disseminated so that the collaboration can actually use them; and they are informative, because, ultimately, they are aimed at improving the outcomes of the collaboration's programs. Empowerment is the core concept, in that the participants are engaged in the process from design to data collection to analysis to dissemination.

In participatory action research, notes Minkler (2000), researchers are "co-learners," rather than teachers: They grapple as equal partners with ethical challenges and the need for research approaches that reflect both scientific and popular perspective. Green et al. (1995) observe that participatory action research is a "systematic investigation," which involves the collaboration of those affected by the matter being studied, for the purposes of education, taking action, or affecting social change. Minkler (2000) makes the case for the special value of participatory action research for evaluating collaboration activities:

- Both participatory action research and collaboration are ground-up, rather than top-down, approaches.
- Both accent the use of democratic participatory processes and social learning about the meaning of health, in order to promote change.
- Both emphasize the strengths of people in communities, including their capacity for problem solving.
- Both tend to be driven by community priorities, rather than those of outside experts.

Finally, Wing (1998) notes that, in order to transform society in support of more fundamental health promotion, a more democratic and ecological approach to scientific study is needed—one in which education of scientists and the public takes place in both directions. Such an approach is time-consuming and filled with challenges, as local communities and outside research collaborators from a variety of sectors attempt to navigate difficult ethical and practical terrain, addressing issues of power and trust, research rigor, and the often conflicting agendas of scientist and citizen (Minkler, 2000).

The first key step to a successful evaluation is *strategic planning* within the collaboration, which will include the development of a mission or goal statement and a list of objectives with time lines. It can also include the strategies to be employed in detailed action plans stating who will do what, when. The strategic plan will flow from some form of needs assessment that identifies relevant issues, barriers, resources, and culturally appropriate ways of dealing with problems. The strategic plan helps the collaboration know where it is going and lays the groundwork for approaching and engaging in the evaluation process.

SO, WHY HIRE AN EVALUATOR?

Often, the most compelling reason is that the funders require that you hire one. Certainly, the advantage of external evaluators is that they bring an objective eye to your collaboration and the evaluation process. However, the collaboration should not rule out that many process evaluations, and even some simple outcome evaluations, can be part of the collaboration's ongoing annual functioning. These do not involve the resources required to hire an external evaluator. As the collaboration completes its own evaluations, evaluation gets built into the collaboration's rhythm, along with running task forces and meetings and producing newsletters.

IF THE COLLABORATION IS IN THE POSITION OF HIRING AN EVALUATOR, THEN WHAT DO ITS MEMBERS LOOK FOR?

Seeking an evaluator who has had experience in evaluating collaborations, and who can provide examples of completed work, makes the process much easier. In many parts of the country, however, a person like that is hard to find. So, what does an organization look for? First, for evaluators who are capable of being sensitive to the local culture (ethnic, racial, political). Second, evaluators need to be able to present information in clear, direct, user-friendly formats. Next, they need to talk *with* the collaboration members and funders, not down to them. Then, they must be able to produce data and reports, in a timely and readable manner, which can be disseminated to collaboration members, to funders, and to the public at large. Finally, an organization wants evaluators who will listen and respond to its needs.

Often, collaborations turn to academic institutions to find evaluators, and many excellent evaluators work within those institutions. However, it is also helpful to look to local market research firms that contract for a service with the business community and produce those services in a timely manner for their customers. The responsiveness to customer needs, which is part of the for-profit market research firm, is one that collaborations should expect from evaluators they hire, no matter what sector they come from—private, public, or academic.

Collaborations need to know that the goal of the evaluation is to improve the collaboration and that the evaluator must be able to provide feedback in a style that can be used to strengthen the collaboration's planning and activities. In every case, the evaluator should apply a utility criterion to the evaluation methods. That is, will this evaluation give the collaboration information that can be used by the collaboration, its members, its funders, and the community? An evaluation does not have much value if it cannot be translated into action. If it won't be used, don't do it (Francisco & Wolff, 1994).

WHAT QUESTIONS SHOULD THE EVALUATION HELP ANSWER?

- *Process evaluation: What activities took place?* This kind of evaluation focuses on the day-to-day activities of your collaboration. Methodologies here may include activity logs, surveys, and interviews. The key variables might involve in-house developments, outside meetings, communications received, community participation, and media coverage. Surveys can be done to rate the importance of feasibility of goals and satisfaction of membership. Process evaluation might also include an analysis of critical events in the development of the collaboration.
- *Outcome evaluation: What was accomplished?* This kind of evaluation focuses on the collaboration's accomplishments. It can include the number and type of changes and policies or practices in the community, as well as the development of new services. It can also be useful to do surveys of self-reported behavior changes and surveys, rating the significance of outcomes achieved. The number of objectives met over time is a useful outcome evaluation tool.
- *Impact evaluation: What were the long-term effects?* This kind of evaluation focuses on the ultimate impacts that the collaboration is having on the community, over and above specific outcomes. The focus here is on statistical indicators. A teen pregnancy collaboration might focus on the pregnancy rate for its locale. Once the results have been collected and reports written, the collaboration must actively engage in a process of dissemination of the findings to allow the community to look at the data, decide what changes are necessary in response to the evaluation findings, and move ahead to change or adapt the strategic plan and the collaboration's activities to reflect the results found in the evaluation.

EVALUATION TOOLS

At the end of this chapter is a series of nine process and outcome evaluation tools, most of which can be easily used by a collaboration on its own, but which can also be part of a repertoire of tools used by an external evaluator with the collaboration. This is by no means a comprehensive collection of all appropriate process and outcome tools for a collaboration. It does represent, however, many tools that have been used by this author in a wide range of collaborations, and have generally been found to pass the utility test. That is, engaging in this evaluation has been useful to the collaboration in re-assessing its position and moving forward in a more effective manner.

Worksheet 1: Annual Satisfaction Surveys for Community Coalitions

A wide range of surveys has been developed for collaborations to use in canvassing the membership on their sense of how well they think the collaboration is doing on a variety of dimensions. This survey was developed by the Work Group at the University of Kansas (Fawcett, Foster, & Francisco, 1997) and judges satisfaction in the following dimensions: planning and implementation, leadership, community involvement in the collaboration, communication, and progress and outcome.

Within the planning and implementation dimension, the survey looks at aspects of the collaboration, such as the vision, planning process, follow-through, strength and competence of staff, and capacity to promote collaborative action. Within the leadership area, it deals with the competence of the collaboration's management, sensitivity to cultural issues, its willingness to engage members in leadership roles, and the degree of trust in the collaboration.

Community involvement evaluates the collaboration's capacity to reach people in key sectors of the community, the participation of community residents, and the diversity of the membership. Communication considers working with the media, and being in touch with members and the broader community. Progress and outcome looks at whether the collaboration is meeting its objectives, generating resources, distributing funds in a fair manner, and contributing to improving community life. Finally, at the end of the survey, a general question is asked about whether the community is better off today because of the collaboration. This format, although very general and subjective, can be very helpful to a collaboration in getting a sense of its members' views of the collaboration and developing action plans to respond to the results.

In some communities where we have administered this instrument, there is a consistent finding that, although leadership is strong, community involvement is not high, especially for community residents. Some collaborations, in response to such findings, have developed active recruiting plans to engage residents in collaboration activities. The advantages of the satisfaction surveys are that they are simple, straightforward, and easy, although they can be somewhat time-consuming to score. It is easy to report the findings and easy for a collaboration to understand what the findings mean, then engage in a process to modify their activities based on the members' perceptions.

The items in each of the categories, and the categories themselves, can be modified to represent specific areas of interest of a given collaboration. The great strength of satisfaction surveys is that they can overcome the excuse of many collaboration members who say, "We don't have the instruments, we don't have time, we don't have the resources to do an evaluation." At least with the satisfaction survey, collaboration members check in with each other on a regular basis about how they think the collaboration is doing. We have seen collaborations implement this survey and successfully use the results to demonstrate to potential funders their seriousness in looking at their progress.

Worksheet 2: Diagnosing Your Coalition: Risk Factors for Participation

This second form is similar to the satisfaction survey, but more detailed, easier to score, and easier to diagnose for remedies. It was developed by Gillian Kaye (1993). In the risk factor diagnosis, Kaye suggests that partnerships look at where they are at risk of discouraging active participation of members, which parts of the collaboration are in good shape, and which could use a tune-up. Each of the items is scored from 1 to 5, and the categories covered include clarity of vision; effectiveness of the initiative's structure; effectiveness of outreach and communication tools and methods; effectiveness of collaboration meetings; opportunities for member responsibility and growth; effectiveness of the partnership's planning and doing; the collaboration's use of research and external resources; the partnership's sense of community; how well the initiative meets needs and provides benefits; and the group's relationship with the elected officials, institutional leaders, and other power players. Kaye has a scoring guideline for each of the sections. This is an easily administered instrument that collaborations can use to look more carefully at a range of internal functions of the collaboration.

Worksheet 3: Assessing Your Collaboration's Commitment to Agency- and Community-Based Approaches

This tool can assist collaborations in assessing their present level of commitment to agency-based and community-based approaches. It can also help the group plan for where they would like to be on these dimensions in the future.

A core belief of collaborations is that they often encourage diverse citizen participation and widespread community ownership. Many collaborations use the words "citizen drive" or "grassroots" in describing the core beliefs of their efforts. Yet, often, when we sit in a room at a collaboration meeting and we look around, we mainly see the faces of the formal community service providers. We know that some of these providers of service are also residents of the community and thus are both residents and formal helpers (although that is not always true). Too often, though, community residents and grassroots organizations are just not at the table.

Chavis and Florin (1990) originally introduced these concepts, using the terms "community-based" and "community development." The community-based approach works with community members primarily as consumers of services and is deficit-oriented. The community development approach works with community members in planning and producing services and builds on a community's strengths. Both approaches have value. They represent two ends of a continuum, and elements of each can be present in any given program. For this assessment tool, we have changed the language to "agency-based" and "community-based," because these terms seem to be easier to understand and to use for communities across the country. For openers, evaluators can look around the room and see who is present, as a first step in assessing which approach they use.

This assessment is best done in small groups of collaboration members, but also can be done by individuals. The scale asks, "Where does your collaboration fall on this dimension? Put an X on the continuum. Where would you like to be in the future? Put an O on the continuum. How can you get to the desired state?" Group discussion on how to reach the desired outcome is encouraged.

This instrument has been especially helpful to collaboration steering committees as they design or reassess their direction and their membership. It allows them to visit or revisit the basic premises of their approach, and to project a new direction for the future, if they wish to change. The content of the instrument is as follows:

- *Approach/Orientation.* An agency-based approach emphasizes the community's weaknesses, and solves the community's problems by addressing its deficits. A community-based approach builds on the community's strengths and assets. The approach involves developing the community's competencies.
- *Definition of the problem.* In an agency-based approach, agencies, government, or outside organizations define the problem for the com-

munity. For example, a state government may make collaboration grants available to the 10 communities with the highest rate of substance abuse. In a community-based approach, the problem is defined by the target community itself. In this approach, the community is asked, or asks itself, "What are our biggest problems and which should we address?"

- *Primary vehicle for creating change.* Agency-based efforts focus on creating individual change through improving services or providing information or education. Community-based efforts aim to build community control and capacity by increasing the community's resources and creating economic and political change.
- *Role of professionals.* Professionals are central to decision making in the agency-based approach, rather than being one of many resources for the community's problem-solving process in the community-based approach.
- *Purpose of participation by target community members and institutions.* In an agency-based initiative, the purpose for participation by the community is to help adapt or adjust services or to disseminate information about existing services. The focus is on the provision of services. In the community-based initiative, the purpose for participation is to increase the community's control and ownership and to improve social conditions in the community.
- *Role of human service agencies and formal helpers.* Human services are the central mechanism for service delivery in the agency-based approach. In the community-based approach, they are one of the many sectors in the community that have been activated to meet the needs of the community.
- *Primary decision makers.* In the agency-based approach, the key decisions are made by agency and government representatives and leaders from business. In the community-based model, the primary decision makers are the informal and local indigenous leaders of the community—the people most affected by the issue being addressed. So, if the community is designing programs for youth, who is making the decisions—the agency personnel or the youth themselves?
- *View of community.* In the agency-based approach, the community is seen as the site of the problem and the community members of the community are seen as the consumers or potential consumers of services. In the community-based approach, the community is seen simply as the place where people live. It is seen subjectively, rather than viewed externally and technically. The agency-based view might be

that this is a community with a high rate of teen pregnancy, but the community-based view can be a concern for Sally, the 16-year-old new mom who lives down the street with her family.

- *Community control of resources.* In the agency-based approach, the community's control of resources (in the community and in the collaboration) is low. A community-based approach ensures that the community's control of all resources is high.
- *Potential for ownership by community members.* In the agency-based approach, community ownership of the process is low, and, in the community-based model, community ownership is higher.

Worksheet 4: Climate Diagnostic Tool: The Six Rs of Participation

This instrument is a helpful way for a collaboration to assess the environment it has created and how hospitable it is to engaging and retaining community members. The instrument is based on research (Kaye & Resnick, 1994) that looked at what key factors of an organization attract citizens to join it and keep citizens engaged in its processes. It turns out that, if an organization is able to provide the "six Rs," it increases the probability that residents of the community will stick with the organization. The six Rs are recognition, respect, role, relationship, reward, and results.

- *Recognition.* People wish to be recognized for their contributions to communities and collaborations. At first, they wish to be recognized by the members of their own groups, then, increasingly, by the members of other groups. Collaboration members wish to be recognized for their efforts and contributions to build a better quality of life for the community and for their special contributions to the workings of the collaboration.
- *Respect.* Everyone wants respect. By participating in community activities, we often seek the respect of our peers. Respect involves an appreciation for people's values, culture, and traditions, and there may not be many settings in a community that can provide that respect for community members. By joining collaborations and other community organizations, people are seeking not only recognition, but also respect for themselves.
- *Role.* We all have the need to feel needed. People want to belong to a group that gives them a meaningful role and in which their unique

contributions can be appreciated. Not everyone is seeking the same role, not everyone wants to be the leader, but everyone wants to feel useful, and collaborations that can provide useful roles to members are much more successful in maintaining membership.

- *Relationships.* Relationships are the heart of the collaboration's work. Often a personal invitation convinces members to join the collaboration. People join for many reasons, among which are: to meet new people, to make new links, and to broaden their base of support and influence. Collaborations draw community members into a wider context of community relationships, which encourage accountability, mutual support, and responsibility.
- *Rewards.* Collaborations attract and maintain members when the rewards of membership outweigh the costs. Not everyone is looking for the same kind of rewards. Collaborations need to identify what the self-interests of the members are, what they are seeking, and how to go about meeting their needs.
- *Results.* Nothing works like results. An organization that cannot deliver the goods will not continue to attract people and resources. All collaboration members come into a meeting with a cost–benefit scale in their heads. They ask, "Is it worth it on a Thursday afternoon at 5:00 to sit for an hour and a half with this group of folks and try to make a change in our community?" The ultimate measure is whether anything gets done. Grassroots community leaders are even tougher on this issue than agency people who are being paid to sit in the room. They are giving up their precious personal time, and they want to know if this is going to make their community better.

This process tool allows a collaboration to assess itself on these six Rs of participation. It suggests that the collaboration members get to understand the definition of the six Rs, then for each of them to ask themselves, for example, What are we doing now as a collaboration to encourage recognition, and what else could we be doing to encourage it? Having done this for all six of the Rs, the collaboration can then develop an action plan that will increase the likelihood that community members will stay with the collaboration and become more active participants.

Worksheet 5: Responsibility Charting

Community collaborations are complex organizational systems with multiple components and multiple actors having some role and responsibility in the collaboration's functioning. Among the key actors are: (1) a *funder* (a foundation; state, local, or federal government; or other source); (2) a *local fiscal agent*, which is the conduit for the dollars, and may even be the employer of the collaboration staff; (3) a *steering committee or board of directors*, which runs the collaboration and provides the leadership; (4) *task forces and task force leaders*, which take on the specific identified issues of the collaboration and do the nitty-gritty work; (5) *staff*, including a director, administrative staff, and program staff, who are often the most visible representatives of the collaboration and those who are able to commit the most time in a given week to collaboration activities; (6) the *collaboration membership at large*, which may meet on a regular basis, or annually, at collaboration meetings; (7) an *evaluator*; (8) *technical assistance providers*; and, of course; (9) the *community at large*, those most affected by the problem: those living in the community.

The strength of collaborations is that they are new organizations and, perhaps, that they are more flexible than many of the long-standing nonprofit organizations in a community. The downside of a collaboration is that, with these many actors and components to it, there can be confusion and conflict or, more often, inaction. This often occurs, because it is not clear which of the components has the ultimate or immediate responsibility for getting something done. Conflicts can arise between steering committees and collaboration directors, between fiscal agents and steering committees, between task forces and steering committees, and between funders and the collaboration as a whole. Consultants working with collaborations across the country have observed virtually every permutation and combination of difficulty among these various components.

So how does a collaboration sort out who has the responsibility to approve activities? Who has the responsibility for developing the alternatives and making these happen? Who needs to be consulted prior to a decision being reached, and who needs to be informed? Responsibility charting, developed by Florin and Chavis (1996), allows a collaboration to chart out the various actors and the various responsibilities in the collaboration and to see what kind of agreement there is about who has what degree of responsibility.

The collaboration members begin the activity by identifying for themselves who are the key actors and placing them in the blank columns across the top. If there are more than five, the collaboration can add a second page and more actors. To complete the form, the collaboration members indicate, for each actor and responsibility, whether the relationship is approval (A), responsible (R), consulted (C), or informed (I). For example, the first responsibility listed might be to determine goals and priorities. The steering committee of the collaboration may take responsibility for determining goals and priorities. They would get an R. It may also be that task forces and the collaboration at large are consulted about this (C), that the lead agency approves it (A), and that the funders are informed about it (I).

After filling in appropriate letters to indicate each actor's role in each responsibility, the collaboration should turn to the next question: How much agreement is there among those filling out the charts? Responsibility charting is most effective when all the parties listed across the top fill out the form. It is helpful to know that, as in the example above, we may think that the funder just wants to be informed, but may feel that it should be able to approve. We may feel that the fiscal agent needs to approve a decision, and they may say, "We don't want any part of that, all we want to do is be informed." The steering committee may feel that it has responsibility for determining goals and priorities, and yet the community groups that meet with the collaboration may feel that the goals and priorities should really come from the community.

Responsibility charting allows for fascinating discussions around these issues. It can promote some conflict, but, more likely, it will identify spots where there is confusion and allow for processes that bring clarity. Responsibility charting takes some time, and compilation of the scores can be complex. It can be done in a process meeting, with all the parties present filling out charts, then putting the results on newsprint in front of the room, for an open discussion.

Worksheet 6: Inclusivity Checklist

Checklist collaborations often declare that one of their goals is to celebrate the diversity within a community, to be inclusive of all members of the community, to be open to the participation of all the sectors in a community. Yet, many collaborations struggle to bring this amount of diversity into their ranks, and they end up being less inclusive than they had hoped.

For other collaborations, the issues of diversity and inclusivity may not be high on their priority list, but may be brought to them by minority members of the community who feel excluded. Too often, we see community collaborations that declare themselves to be open to all members of the community, but instead represent the majority, the formal structure, the power brokers, rather than the community at large or those representing smaller minority groups.

The inclusivity checklist is an instrument that allows a collaboration to do an internal process assessment about diversity and inclusivity. It gives collaboration members the opportunity to analyze the issues of inclusivity and diversity across a wide range of their collaboration activities. The easiest way for a group to look at the issue is to look around a room at a collaboration meeting or a steering committee meeting and ask how diverse they are in terms of race, gender, and/or ethnicity. More deeply, however, a group can look at such questions as where resources are distributed, who speaks, what are the group's stated goals and objectives, and what does the group do to welcome and encourage members from various groups in the community. The inclusivity checklist, developed by Rosenthal (1997), helps a collaboration make that assessment.

Worksheet 7: Task Force Evaluation and Resource Allocation

Frequently, collaborations function by identifying issues and assigning each to a smaller group made up of key people concerned about a given issue and able to make a difference on it. These subgroups are often called work groups, task forces, or study action groups. Often, in collaborations, these task forces are created and can have a life of their own, continuing for many years, regardless of how effective they are. The rule seems to be: "If you create a task force, it is a task force for life."

So, how does a collaboration deal with this? Hathaway (2001a, 2001b, 2001c), of the Lower Outer Cape Community Collaboration, along with the collaboration's steering committee, developed a Task Force Evaluation and Resource Allocation Process, which is used annually by the steering committee to evaluate the task forces and to allocate resources to the task forces, based on the assessment. The process starts with the task force identifying its members, its goal, and its objectives, including the activities to achieve the goal and the target dates. The task force then requests resources from the collaboration to support its activities. The resources may include staff who will chair the meeting, mail the minutes, and evaluate progress and outcome, as well as any funding resources for programs.

The request goes to the steering committee, which then asks a series of questions, including: Does the task force address the mission of the collaboration? Which goals of the collaboration does it support? Will allocating resources to the task force detract from the core services of the collaboration? How representative is the task force? Is the goal achievable? What is the likely disposition of the task force in the future? Are members of the task force providing resources to support the task force's operation? If additional funds are needed, what potential resources exist? The collaboration steering committee then decides whether or not to provide support in response to the requests made by the task force.

This is an extremely simple process evaluation form to use within collaborations. In my experience, rarely do collaborations evaluate their own task forces. This process leads to an increase of effectiveness and accountability of task forces and clarification of the relationship of the steering committee to its task forces.

Worksheet 8: Sustainability Benchmarks

This tool was developed by the Center for Collaborative Planning (2000) for the Community Partnerships for Healthy Children (CPHC) initiative, based on the work of Wolff (1994), to assess multiple levels of attempts to sustain collaboration efforts. This approach to sustainability of collaborations looks at four possible avenues for sustaining collaborations: *fundraising and incorporation, institutionalizing the effort, policy change,* and *mobilizing the community.* The Center for Collaborative Planning expanded those four concepts into a usable instrument that allows a collaboration to ask itself how it is doing in each of the sustainability benchmarks.

For each of the benchmarks, the collaboration is asked a range of key questions that are meant to help assess their sustainability potential. It is an internal process evaluation of how well the collaboration is doing in trying to plan for sustainability in all four areas. As stated by CPHC, the areas are mobilizing community residents who are committed to sustaining the efforts; creating policy and systems change at local, regional, and state levels; spinning off or institutionalizing effective strategies or programs; and successfully raising funds and/or proceeding with incorporation to sustain the core functioning of the collaboration.

Having answered the four sets of questions, the collaboration then has an overview of the viability of its sustainability plan and is engaged in a community process that broadens the buy-in and concern around the issues of sustainability.

Worksheet 9: Annual Reports

Some of these instruments touch on some aspects of collaboration outcome, but the simplest tool, and one not used nearly enough by collaborations, is simply to issue an annual report of the collaboration's activities. Such a report can begin with a review of its missions, goals, and structure, then summarize the various activities—usually task forces and objectives for the year, task force activities, and the outcomes.

An example of such an annual report from the Lower Outer Cape Community Collaboration (Hathaway, 2001b) is provided here, as the final tool in this set, and many collaborations have used similar approaches. The process of putting together this type of an annual report implies a number of things: that the collaboration has clear mission goals and objectives for its overall functioning; that each of its task forces is set up to work within those mission goals and objectives; that each task force itself has a set of goals, objectives, activities, and outcomes for a given year; and that, at least on an annual basis, someone is collecting and listing those activities and outcomes, and there is a system in place for doing so.

Although this may sound simplistic, few collaborations actually do this. Indeed, many of the outcomes of collaborations are never noted, never celebrated, and the collaboration does not get credit for them. Those who do promote and circulate their findings in a form, such as an annual report, make their members feel proud of their work and able to share their outcomes with others.

ACKNOWLEDGMENTS

The author wishes to thank Megan Howe and Suzanne Cashman for their assistance in the creation of this chapter. The evaluation tools in this chapter are used with their creators' permission; the creators retain the rights to the materials.

INDEX TO COLLABORATION EVALUATION WORKSHEETS

Worksheet 1

Annual Satisfaction Survey for Community Coalitions*

Dear Coalition Member:

The purpose of the attached consumer satisfaction questionnaire is to get your feedback on how well this coalition is doing. As you know, this coalition's mission is to . . . (complete this.)

Please complete each question by circling the number that best shows your satisfaction with that aspect of the coalition. We welcome additional comments and suggestions you have for improving this coalition.

To protect anonymity, please use the enclosed envelope to return your completed questionnaire to our coalition's evaluators, the (complete name of group).

Thanks in advance for your valuable advice and feedback.

Best regards,

OVERALL APPROVAL RATING:

Is the community better off today because of this coalition? (please check one)
    Yes___   No___

Overall comments and suggestions for improvement:

Thanks for your valuable feedback. Please use the attached envelope to return the completed questionnaire to:

> **Instructions:**
> *We welcome your feedback on how well this coalition is doing. For each item, please circle the number that best shows your satisfaction with that aspect of the coalition. Provide additional comments if you wish.*

---

*Fawcett, S., Foster, D., & Francisco, V. (1997). Monitoring and evaluation of coalition activities and success. In G. Kaye & T. Wolff (Eds.), *From the ground up: A workbook on coalition building and community development* (pp. 163–185). Amherst, MA: AHEC/ Community Partners.

Planning and Implementation:

		very dissatisfied				very satisfied
1.	Clarity of the vision for where the coalition should be going	1	2	3	4	5
2.	Planning process used to prepare the coalition's objectives	1	2	3	4	5
3.	Follow-through on coalition activities	1	2	3	4	5
4.	Strength and competence of staff	1	2	3	4	5
5.	Efforts to promote collaborative action	1	2	3	4	5
6.	Processes used to assess the community's needs	1	2	3	4	5
7.	Training and technical assistance provided by staff	1	2	3	4	5

Comments:

Leadership:

		very dissatisfied				very satisfied
8.	Strength and competence of coalition leadership	1	2	3	4	5
9.	Sensitivity to cultural issues	1	2	3	4	5
10.	Opportunities for coalition members to take leadership roles	1	2	3	4	5
11.	Willingness of members to take leadership roles	1	2	3	4	5
12.	Trust that coalition members afford each other	1	2	3	4	5

Comments:

Community Involvement in the Coalition:

		very dissatisfied				very satisfied
13.	Participation of influential people from key sectors of the community	1	2	3	4	. 5
14.	Participation of community residents	1	2	3	4	5

15.	Diversity of coalition members	1	2	3	4	5
16.	Help given the community in meeting its needs	1	2	3	4	5
17.	Help given community groups to become better able to address and resolve their concerns	1	2	3	4	5
18.	Efforts in getting funding for community programs	1	2	3	4	5

Comments:

Communication:

		very dissatisfied				very satisfied
19.	Use of the media to promote awareness of the coalition's goals, actions, and accomplishments	1	2	3	4	5
20.	Communication among members of the coalition	1	2	3	4	5
21.	Communication between the coalition and the broader community	1	2	3	4	5
22.	Extent to which coalition members are listened to and heard	1	2	3	4	5
23.	Working relationships established with elected officials	1	2	3	4	5
24.	Information provided on issues and available resources	1	2	3	4	5

Comments:

Progress and Outcome:

		very dissatisfied				very satisfied
25.	Progress in meeting the coalition's objectives	1	2	3	4	5
26.	Success in generating resources for the coalition	1	2	3	4	5
27.	Fairness with which funds and opportunities are distributed	1	2	3	4	5
28.	Capacity of members to give support to each other	1	2	3	4	5

29. Capacity of the coalition and its members to advocate effectively   1   2   3   4   5

30. Coalition's contribution to improving health and human services in the community   1   2   3   4   5

Comments:

Worksheet 2

Diagnosing Your Coalition: Risk Factors for Participation*

WHY? WHY? WHY?

Why do some members come to every meeting of the coalition and some won't even come to one?

Why are some families so active while others won't even take the time to fill out a survey?

There is no simple or quick answer. But we do know there are a lot of factors that influence why residents and families will and won't get involved in your coalition. Some of these factors are a little harder for the coalition to tackle, such as economic problems in the family and serious lack of time.

BUT ...

You can control one of the most important participation factors: YOUR COALITION! Yes, it's true. Many different parts of a coalition's functioning can encourage or discourage participation! Your coalition might be "at risk" of being a participation discourager and you don't even know it.

One of the important roles of a leader is to step back every once in a while and look, with a critical eye, at how the coalition is working:

- Are all of the coalition's "building blocks" in place to make it a strong coalition?
- Do things get done in a way that encourages members and others to be active and have "ownership" of the coalition?

Use this COALITION RISK FACTOR diagnosis to find out which parts of your coalition are "at risk" of discouraging active participation from members and nonmembers and could use a tune-up, and which parts are humming along. The results may surprise you!

Put a number (based on the 1–5 scale that follows) in the bubble that corresponds to each question. Total up your score at the end of each numbered

---

*Kaye, G. (1993). *Diagnosing your coalition: Risk factors for participation*. Brooklyn, NY: Community Development Consultants.

section and again at the end on the "Diagnosis Score Sheet." Check out your coalition's diagnosis!

NOTE: You'll notice that all of the statements on this form are written in the "positive." But it's more important that you be honest than that your coalition sound "perfect." NO COALITION IS PERFECT!!

RATE THE FOLLOWING PARTS OF YOUR COALITION, USING THE SCALE BELOW:

Strong/Always				Weak/Never
5	4	3	2	1

1. *The Clarity of Your Coalition's Vision and Goals*
    A.   The coalition's vision takes into account what is happening in the community. ○
    B.   The vision and goals are written down. ○
    C.   Residents and institutions are all aware of the vision and goals of the coalition. ○
    D.   The coalition periodically reevaluates and updates its vision and goals. ○
    E.   The activities of the coalition are evaluated in relation to the vision and goals of the coalition. ○

Total #1 ____

NOTES:

2. *The Effectiveness of Your Coalition Structure*
    A.   The coalition has a regular meeting cycle that members can expect. ○
    B.   The coalition has active committees. ○
    C.   All of the members have copies of the by-laws. ○
    D.   The executive board and committees communicate regularly. ○
    E.   The executive board meets on a regular basis with good attendance. ○

Total #2 ____

NOTES:

3. *The Effectiveness of Your Outreach & Communication: Tools &*
    Methods
    A. The coalition has a newsletter or another method of com- ◯
        munication that keeps the school community regularly
        updated and informed about its activities.
    B. The coalition uses a survey or another method to collect ◯
        information about members' interests, needs, and con-
        cerns.
    C. The survey results are always published and used to guide ◯
        the coalition's projects.
    D. The survey is conducted every year or so, because the ◯
        community and residents change.
    E. The coalition "goes to where members are" to do out- ◯
        reach, including where people live, shop, and work.

                                                       Total #3 ____

NOTES:

4. *The Effectiveness of Coalition Meetings*
    A. Members feel free to speak at a meeting without fear of ◯
        being attacked.
    B. The coalition advertises its meetings with sufficient notice ◯
        by sending agendas and flyers out in advance.
    C. Child care and translation are provided at meetings when ◯
        needed.
    D. The work of the meeting, as outlined in the agenda, gets ◯
        accomplished because meetings start and end on time.
    E. The meetings are held in central, convenient, and comfort- ◯
        able places and at convenient times for all members.

                                                       Total #4 ____

NOTES:

5. *Opportunities for Member Responsibility and Growth*
    A. The coalition makes a conscious effort to develop new ◯
        leaders.
    B. Training and support are offered to new leaders, as well ◯
        as to the more experienced leaders (by the coalition or
        through outside agencies).
    C. A "buddy system" matches less experienced members ◯

with leaders to help them learn jobs and make contacts.
D.   Committees are given serious work to do.
E.   Leadership responsibilities are shared in the coalition; that is, chairing a meeting is a job that rotates.

Total #5 ____

NOTES:

6.   *The Coalition's Effectiveness in Doing Projects (Planning, Implementing, and Evaluating)*
   A.   At the beginning of each new year, the coalition develops a plan that includes goals and activities that it wants to accomplish during the year.
   B.   The plans are based, at least in part, on information collected from surveys of members.
   C.   After each activity or project, the leadership or the committee evaluates how it went, in order to learn from the experience.
   D.   The coalition always organizes visible projects that make a difference to members.
   E.   When projects are undertaken, action plans, which identify tasks, who will do what, and target dates, are developed.

Total #6 ____

NOTES:

7.   *Your Coalition's Use of Research/External Resources*
   A.   The coalition works within the community on common issues and with citywide coalitions that work on critical community concerns.
   B.   The coalition utilizes resources and information on other coalitions that can help the community, that is, training workshops on environmental organizing.
   C.   The coalition stays on top of issues affecting communities across the city and state.
   D.   Outside speakers come to meetings to speak on topics of interest to members.
   E.   When the coalition wants to work on an issue, leaders know where to go to get necessary information, that is, statistics, forms, and so on.

Total #7 ____

NOTES:

8. *Your Coalition's Sense of Community*
    A. The coalition builds social time into the meetings, so that ◯ people can talk informally and build a sense of community.
    B. The coalition plans fun social activities.   ◯
    C. Everyone in the coalition is treated equally.   ◯
    D. All contributions from members, large and small, are   ◯ recognized and rewarded.
    E. All residents are made to feel welcome in the coalition,   ◯ regardless of income, race, gender, or education level.

                                                      Total #8 ____

NOTES:

9. *How Well the Coalition Meets Needs and Provides Benefits*
    A. Resource lists and important contacts are regularly made   ◯ available to members.
    B. Workshops are held with "experts" who can provide con-   ◯ crete services to members.
    C. The coalition helps members with issues of individual   ◯ need.
    D. If a survey of the members indicated that personal issues   ◯ (such as child care or landlord/tenant problems) were getting in the way of residents' involvement, the coalition would respond to those issues.
    E. The coalition holds meetings and workshops where resi-   ◯ dents can meet elected officials and city service personnel, to voice their opinions and learn about resources and programs in the community.

                                                      Total #9 ____

NOTES:

10. *The Coalition's Relationship With Elected Officials, Institutional Leaders, and Other Power Players*
    A. The coalition leaders know how to negotiate with "power   ◯ players," such as elected officials and institutional leaders, and how to successfully "win" on issues of concern to members.

B. The coalition has regular representatives who attend important ◯ community meetings.

C. Leaders and members of the coalition understand the lines of ◯ authority, decision-making power, responsibilities, and other aspects of the "power structure" of the community.

D. The coalition meets with officials on a regular basis about the ◯ issues that concern members.

E. The coalition participates in citywide activities and demonstra- ◯ tions that focus on community issues.

Total #10 _____

NOTES:

DIAGNOSIS SCORE SHEET

Fill out this score sheet using the *total numbers* from each section of the
Coalition Diagnosis.

1. VISION/SENSE OF PURPOSE   TOTAL #1:
2. COALITION STRUCTURE   TOTAL #2:
3. OUTREACH/COMMUNICATION   TOTAL #3:
4. COALITION MEETINGS   TOTAL #4:
5. MEMBER RESPONSIBILITY/GROWTH   TOTAL #5:
6. DOING PROJECTS   TOTAL #6:
7. RESEARCH/EXTERNAL RESOURCES   TOTAL #7:
8. SENSE OF COMMUNITY   TOTAL #8:
9. NEEDS AND BENEFITS   TOTAL #9:
10. RELATIONSHIP WITH POWER PLAYERS   TOTAL #10:

FINAL SCORE FOR DIAGNOSIS: ____

YOUR COALITION'S DIAGNOSIS

FOR EACH SECTION, FOLLOW THE GUIDELINES BELOW:

IF YOU SCORED BETWEEN:

5 and 15   **Check-up time!!** You may need an "overhaul" in this area.

15 and 20   **Watch out!!** It's time for a "tune-up" to get everything in
good working order.

20 and 25   **Congratulations!!** You're running smoothly and all systems
are go! Keep up the good work!

Worksheet 3

Assessing Your Collaboration's Commitment to Agency-Based and Community-Based Approaches*

> ### Instructions:
>
> Mark an "X" on the continuum for where you currently are.
> Mark an "O" on the continuum for where you would like to be.

Issues	Agency-Based	Continuum	Community-Based
Approach/orientation	Weakness/deficit solve problems	_____	Strength/Competence capacity
Definition of problem	By agencies, government, or outside	_____	By target community
Primary vehicles for healthy promotion and change	Education, improved services, lifestyle change, food availability, media	_____	Building community control, increasing community resources and capacity, and economic structure
Role of professionals	Key, central to decision making	_____	Resource
Role of participation by target community members and institutions	Providing better services, increasing consumption and support	_____	To increase target community control and social structure
Role of human service agencies and formal	Central mechanism for service delivery	_____	One of many systems activated to respond to the needs of a target community members

*Chavis, E., & Florin, P. (1990). *Community participation and substance abuse prevention: Rationale, concepts and mechanisms.* County of Santa Clara, CA: Bureau of Drug Abuse Services.

Primary decision makers	Agency representatives, business leaders, government representatives, "appointed" community leaders	————	By target community leaders
View of community development consultants	Broad, site of the problem technically and externally defined, consumers	————	Specific, targeted, source of solution, internally defined, subjective, a place to live
Target community control of resources	Low	————	High
Potential for ownership by target community members	Low	————	High

Worksheet 4

Climate Diagnostic Tool: The Six Rs of Participation*

> *Instructions:*
> Please rate how well your organization/collaboration/initiative does the following, using the scale below. Tabulate your scores for each section. (*For established groups, have each individual fill out the diagnostic, then compare your answers and attempt to come up with a group diagnostic. For new groups, prioritize the items in each section, then discuss: (a) What do you currently have the capacity to do? and (b) What do you need to develop the capacity to do?*)

1	2	3	4	5	6
Poor	Fair	Average	Good	Excellent	N/A

I. Recognition

People want to be recognized for their leadership to serve the members of their communities and organizations. We all want to be recognized, initially by the members of our own groups and then by members of other groups, for our personal contribution to efforts to build a better quality of life.

Does your organization/collaboration:

❑ Regularly praise members or individuals for work they have done, through awards, dinners, or other public events?

❑ Regularly praise members or individuals for work they have done, even small tasks by recognizing them in meetings and on occasions when others are present?

❑ Contact members or individuals after they have completed a task or contributed to an event or program and privately thank them?

❑ Use a newsletter or other written communication tool to praise and recognize member or individual contributions?

❑ SCORE *(for this section)*

---

*Kaye, G., & Resnick, I. (1994). *Climate Diagnostic Tool*. Brooklyn, NY: Community Development Consultants.

II. Respect

Everyone wants respect. By joining in community activities, we seek the respect of our peers. People often find that their values, culture, or traditions are not respected in the work place or community. People seek recognition and respect for themselves and their values by joining community organizations and initiatives.

Does your organization/collaboration:

❑ Thoughtfully delegate tasks, making sure that members' and individuals' skills and strengths are being used?

❑ Provide translators or translated materials for members or individuals who do not speak English as their first language?

❑ Include celebrations and traditions that reflect the diversity of your membership and/or community?

❑ Reflect the diversity of your membership and/or community, through the foods and refreshments you share at meetings, and other events?

❑ Provide child care at meetings and/or dinner at evening meetings, so that people with families and children can participate equally?

❑ Hold your meetings at times other than during the 9–5 workday, so that people who work or go to school during those hours and cannot take time off can attend?

❑ Listen to and acknowledge the contribution of all members?

❑ SCORE *(for this section)*

III. Role

We all need to feel needed. It is a cliché, but it is true. We want to belong to a group that gives us an important role, and where our unique contribution can be appreciated. Not everyone searches for the same role. But groups must find a role for everyone, if they expect to maintain engagement.

Does your organization/collaboration:

❑ Provide the same kinds of roles for professionals and nonprofessionals with the same responsibility and power?

❑ Delegate tasks to grassroots members and individuals that involve contacts with important stakeholders and others with power?

❑ Ask members and individuals what kind of roles they would like to play in the organization/collaboration?

❑ Dedicate some portion of time to working with grassroots members and individuals to develop their skills to accomplish these tasks and play these roles?

❑ SCORE *(for this section)*

IV. Relationship

Organizations are organized networks of relationships. It is often a personal invitation that convinces us to join an organization. People join organizations for personal reasons, to make new friends, and for the public reason to broaden a base of support and/or influence. Organizations draw us into a wider context of community relationships that encourage accountability, mutual support, and responsibility.

Does your organization/collaboration:

❑ Regularly provide opportunities for socializing before and after meetings?

❑ Provide opportunities for members and individuals to formally network with each other around common interests?

❑ Provide opportunities for grassroots members and individuals to meet with powerful stakeholders who have access to, and who may or may not be part of your organization?

❑ Provide opportunities for individuals to work together as partners on projects and tasks?

❑ SCORE *(for this section)*

V. Reward

Organizations and coalitions attract new members and maintain old members, when the rewards of membership outweigh the costs. Of course, not everyone is looking for the same kind of rewards.

Does your organization/collaboration:

❑ Work to identify the public and private rewards that respond to the self-interests of members and individuals? In other words, does it try to understand what people want out of their involvement and try to meet their self-interest?

❏   Provide the same information and access to funding opportunities to
    all members and individuals who are involved with the organization/
    collaboration?
❏   Provide other resources and/or referrals to members and individuals
    involved with the organization/collaboration that matter to them?
❏   Create opportunities for members to share information and other re-
    sources among themselves in special interest committees or some other
    way?

❏ SCORE *(for this section)*

VI.   Results

Nothing works like results! An organization or initiative needs to be able to
"deliver the goods."

Does your organization/collaboration:

❏   Have short-term goals and projects that show immediate results on
    issues that matter to grassroots members and individuals?
❏   Have long-term goals and projects that will create meaningful change?
❏   Welcome members and individuals who have specific concerns that
    may not fit directly into your long-term agenda, but may fit indirectly
    and have the support of others in the community?
❏   Use short-term victories as a way to build your base of membership
    or involvement in the community?

❏ SCORE *(for this section)*

When you have completed the diagnostic, score the results. Using the handout
provided, discuss the results with your team and facilitator, and answer the
following questions:

•   What do we do well?
•   What more can we do in each of these areas?

Climate Diagnostic Score Sheet

Use the guidelines below to help your group identify areas that need to be
strengthened. While there is no "magic bullet" for getting citizens engaged

and keeping them at the table, these "Six Rs" are a good guide to understanding what will keep people involved.

If you've scored in the lower numbers, take some time to reflect on what you could be doing differently to improve your process. If you've scored in the middle numbers, don't just move on and assume you're doing all you can. Keep trying to improve your work in these areas. If you've scored in the higher numbers, you should feel positive about the effort you are putting in to making your initiative, collaboration, or organization a welcoming place for citizens to be active partners. Remember, though, that there is always work to be done to continue to improve and grow.

Section I: Recognition

If you scored:

4–9   Take a hard look at what you are doing or not doing to satisfy people's need for recognition. Can you provide more opportunities for praising members or individuals and their contributions? Do you have a newsletter? Create one! Do you focus specific time and attention on recognizing members and other individuals?

10–15   You're on your way, but not there yet. You're still at risk for discouraging participation. Keep trying to think of new ideas and make recognizing people a regular part of your dialogue and contact with members and others.

25–35   Good job. You understand the value and importance of recognizing folks for their contributions and are succeeding in making this an active part of how your organization, initiative, or collaboration operates. Keep the focus!

Section II: Respect

If you scored:

7–15   Take a hard look at how you offer folks the opportunity to be respected for their involvement. Do you need to delegate better so that you are empowering folks, rather than intimidating them with tasks they are not ready to take on? Are you doing what you can to recognize and welcome diversity in your membership or in the community? Do your meetings happen on a "service provider" schedule, making it difficult for other community members to get involved?

16–24   You're on your way, but not there yet. Think about how you present yourselves to the community. Is your initiative, organization, or collaboration a place where diverse people feel welcome and included? Do you give off the impression that only "professionals" have a seat at the table? Keep trying to identify what the community needs to feel respected and work this into your day-to-day operations.

25–35   Good job. You understand the value and importance of making people feel they are respected for their differences, circumstances, and the unique skills and contributions they bring. You are succeeding in making this an active part of how your organization, initiative, or collaboration operates. Keep the focus!

Section III: Role

If you scored:

4–9   Take a hard look at whether you are providing real and valuable roles for citizens, not just "professionals," in your work. Are you working at developing the leadership skills some grassroots folks may need to take on, roles that have value and substance? Do you fairly delegate tasks or just do what's easiest? Are you actively trying to identify what roles will have meaning to folks who are interested in joining you, but may not know exactly how they can fit in to your work?

10–15   You're on your way, but not there yet. Focus time on developing leadership skills and abilities among the "nonprofessionals" who are interested in working with you, and work hard at understanding what roles folks want to play. Brush up on your own delegating skills and make sure delegating is done fairly and well.

15–20   Good job. You understand the value and importance of providing real and valuable roles for all members and individuals who want to work with you in your efforts and how to make this happen. Keep the focus!

Section IV: Relationships

If you scored:

4–9   Take a hard look at whether you are providing enough and the right kinds of opportunities for folks to network and build relationships, inside and outside your organization, collaboration, or initiative. Do you have dinners, recreational activities, or other socializing opportunities built into your operations? Do you provide occasions for "regular" folks and "power players" to meet and work or talk together?

10–15   You're on your way, but not there yet. Work to understand the value of social time, relationship building and networking to potential and existing community members and others who want to work with you and build these experiences into your day-to-day work. Having the opportunity to work with folks who have like agendas and issues is critical for keeping people involved and creating a climate for involvement.

15–20   Good job. You understand the value and importance of promoting and building relationships as a key part of your organization, initiative, or collaboration's operating and are providing opportunities for folks to form relationships with each other and with decision makers and other "power players." Keep the focus.

Section V: Reward

If you scored:

4–9   Take a hard look at whether you are providing rewards for people's involvement that outweigh the costs of working with you. Are you taking the important time to identify the self-interest of members and individuals and working with this information to provide rewards and incentives for getting involved? Is everyone getting the same information and resources that will make involvement of benefit to their organizations, families, and/or other interests?

10–15   You're on your way, but not there yet. Can you do anything else to better understand the self-interest of members and others who want to work with you and to match this self-interest with work in your initiative, organization, or collaboration? Providing resources and allowing folks to work on what interests them is an important part of creating a climate for involvement.

15–20   Good job. You understand the value and importance of providing rewards for people's involvement and matching self-interest with the activities and work of your organization, initiative, or collaboration. Keep the focus.

Section VI: Results

If you scored:

4–9   Take a hard look at how result-focused your organization, collaboration, or initiative is in its work. Are you providing space for short-term meaningful "wins" or just focused on long-term projects that require a lot of time and planning? Are you too focused on short-term "wins" and don't have any long-term vision for real change? Are you open to other ideas from community members that matter to the community, or are you too rigid about your agenda?

10–15 You're on your way, but not there yet. Can you create a better balance between short-term meaningful victories and long-term systems change? Building a base of community involvement means being open to taking on issues the community sees as critical, which may not be exactly on your agenda.

15–20 Good job. You understand the value and importance of results, short-term and long-term, for building involvement and keeping members and others on board and can balance short-term victories with long-term systems change. Keep the focus.

Worksheet 5

Responsibility Charting*

While clarity can be promoted through general structural and procedural means, the complexity of work groups, such as collaborations, often makes even more detailed specification necessary. A useful tool for this purpose is responsibility charting. This tool helps to develop mutual understanding among various actors with respect to various tasks and decision-making activities.

Below is a sample responsibility chart. You may make additions either to the actors or tasks/decisions column. Simply place the appropriate letter within each box to indicate the specific role of each actor. For example, say the project director and other staff are responsible for planning methods for program delivery. Furthermore, the steering committee must be consulted on methods prior to a vote of approval by the entire collaboration, while a separate board for the project need only be informed by the project director.

The responsibility chart for this situation would look as follows:

	Project Director	Staff	Council	Sterring Committee	Board
Plan models (methods) for program delivery	R	R	A	C	I

Responsibility Chart

Codes

A = *Approve.* Must sign off or veto before implementation or select from options developed by **R** role.

R = *Responsible.* Takes initiative in areas, develops alternatives, makes recommendation.

C = *Consulted.* Must be consulted prior to decision being reached, but has no veto power.

I = *Informed.* Must be notified after a decision, but before public announcement. Needs to know outcome for other related tasks, but need not give input.

---

*Florin, P., & Chavis, D. (1996). *Responsibility charting.* Gaithersburg, MD: Association for the Study and Development of Community.

Analysis of Your Responsibility Chart

A complete analysis of responsibility charting should be done in collaboration with all important actors. Here, a quick look at the codes in your chart can address the following questions:

A.   Do too many "Don't knows" indicate the need for more structural and procedural specification?

B.   Do the project directors have too many responsibilities? This not only sets the project director up for "burnout," but also prevents the fullest development of participation and leadership from other participants.

C.   Is there a sufficient level of participation by the collaboration members to promote "ownership" of decisions?

D.   How can you use the structure and procedures of your collaboration (e.g., delegating to subcommittees, rotating leadership) to promote higher levels of participation?

E.   Can you "cluster" various tasks/decisions according to planning and policy, implementation, and day-to-day administrative categories?

F.   What other agencies/organizations besides those in the collaboration, should be kept informed of your activities? How will they be so informed?

The responsibility chart itself could be shared and approved by the various committees and boards.

Responsibility Chart
Actors

1.	Determine goals/priorities						
2.	Suggest alternatives—strategies and programs						
3.	Decide on programs for implementation						
4.	Identify resources for programs						
5.	Community and public relations						
6.	Program administration						
7.	Recruit new collaboration members						
8.	Chair meetings						
9.	Prepare agendas						
10.	Staff hiring						
11.	Develop personnel policies						
12.	Recruit volunteers						
13.	Maintain communications						
14.	Prepare budget						
15.	Approve budget						
16.	Purchases						
17.	Collaboration leadership						
18.	Decision making						
19.							
20.							

Worksheet 6

Inclusivity Checklist*

> *Instructions:*
> *Use this Inclusivity Checklist to measure how prepared your coalition is for multicultural work and to identify areas for improvement. Place a check mark in the box next to each statement that applies to your group. If you cannot put a check in the box, this may indicate an area for change.*

❑ The leadership of our coalition is multiracial and multicultural.

❑ We make special efforts to cultivate new leaders, particularly women and people of color.

❑ Our mission, operations, and products reflect the contributions of diverse cultural and social groups.

❑ We are committed to fighting social oppression within the coalition and in our work in the community.

❑ Members of diverse cultural and social groups are full participants in all aspects of our coalition's work.

❑ Meetings are not dominated by speakers from any one group.

❑ All segments of our community are represented in decision making.

❑ We are sensitive to and aware of different religious and cultural holidays, customs, recreation, and food preferences.

❑ We communicate clearly, and people of different cultures feel comfortable sharing their opinions and participating in meetings.

❑ We prohibit the use of stereotypes and prejudicial comments.

❑ Ethnic, racial, and sexual slurs or jokes are not welcome.

---

*Rosenthal, B. (1997). Multicultural issues in coalitions. In Kaye, G., & Wolff, T. (Eds.), *From the ground up: A workbook on coalition building and community development.* Amherst, MA: AHEC/Community Partners.

Worksheet 7

Task Force Evaluation and Resource Allocation*

> **Instructions:**
> The task force should fill out the first page of this two-page evaluation, as part of an annual evaluation process. After agreeing on responses and resource requests as a group, the task force should pass the form to the coalition's steering committee for resource allocation assessment (page 2).

Task Force:

Date Formed:

Purpose:

Current Task Force Members (name and affiliation): _____
   Chair:

Goal (the work of this Task Force will be done when):

Objectives/activities to achieve goal and target dates:

Resources to support Task Force—Indicate person or organization that will provide each service and check those requested from Coalition:

Chair meetings (schedule, set agenda, facilitate meetings)	Participate in meetings
Type and mail minutes and other correspondence	Evaluate progress and outcomes
Send meeting notices and make follow-up calls	Promote work and activities of Task Force
Carry out activities of Task Force (Specify)	Other (Specify)

Do you anticipate that additional funds will be needed to reach the goal?

Other considerations:

1. Does this Task Force address the mission of the coalition to improve the quality of life for those living in the program area?

---

*Hathaway, B. L. (1998). *Task force evaluation and resource allocation.* Orleans, MA: Lower/Outer Cape Community Coalition.

2. Which goal(s) does it support?
    ❏ To mobilize and maintain broad-based community development and collaboration problem-solving initiatives around health and human services.
    ❏ To ensure the availability of and access to basic opportunities and services.
    ❏ To provide leadership in developing policies, practices, and programs that are effective, responsive, and accountable to those they serve.
3. Will allocating resources to this Task Force detract from the core services?
4. Is there a cross-section of the community represented on the Task Force?
        If no, who else should be represented?
5. Is the goal achievable?
6. What is the likely disposition of this Task Force in the future?
7. Are members providing resources to support the Task Force?
8. If additional funds will be needed, what potential sources exist?
9. Other

Coalition support to be provided:
❏ None at this time
❏ Chair meetings (schedule, set agenda, facilitate meetings)
❏ Participate in meetings
❏ Type and mail minutes and other correspondence
❏ Send meeting notices and make follow-up calls
❏ Promote work and activities of Task Force
❏ Evaluate progress and outcomes
❏ Carry out activities of Task Force (specify):
❏ Other (specify):

Worksheet 8

Sustainability Benchmarks*

Instructions

1. Review the five Sustainability Benchmarks that follow.
2. With coalition membership, discuss each benchmark, to determine present strengths and challenges and possible actions.
3. Respond to each benchmark in 1–2 pages of narrative. Note that the key questions are meant to aid you in your thinking. **You do not need to answer each question directly.**
4. Remember that this process is meant to help you assess your sustainability potential. The actions you identify will go into your sustainability plan.
5. We hope you will use this tool for a thoughtful and honest assessment and that your narrative reflects this honesty. In that way, training and technical assistance can be tailored for the next year.

Note: These benchmarks and key questions can be tailored to your organization's specific needs and activities. Use what follows as a guide.

I   **The collaboration has mobilized community residents who are committed to sustaining efforts to improve the community.**

A collaboration successful at this sustainability strategy understands that the gifts, talents, skills, and capacities of individuals are essential building blocks for healthy communities. In addition, a mobilized citizenry that feels ownership of, and contributes to, collaborative efforts is key to long-term sustainability.

(Please respond in 1–2 pages. Describe your strengths, challenges, and proposed actions. The Key Questions are to aid you in thinking about the benchmark.)

---

*Center for Collaborative Planning (2000). *Sustainability Benchmarks*. Sacramento, CA: Author.

Key Questions:
A. How has your collaboration identified the gifts, talents, skills, and capacities of community residents?
B. How has your collaboration provided opportunities for these gifts and capacities to be contributed?
C. How are these gifts and capacities being used to sustain collaboration efforts?
D. How has your collaboration acknowledged and celebrated contributions that have been made?

II. **The collaboration is sustaining its efforts to improve the community through policy and systems change at the local, regional, and state level.**

A collaboration successful at this sustainability strategy views a mobilized local citizenry as an effective constituency to improve the community. The collaboration has built its own capacity and the capacity of a mobilized citizenry to understand how policy is made and influenced and to develop and implement policy and systems change strategies to improve the community.

(Please respond in 1–2 pages. Describe your strengths, challenges, and proposed actions. The Key Questions are to aid you in thinking about this benchmark.)

Key Questions:
A. How has the collaboration built its own capacity, and the capacity of community members, to understand how policy and systems change occurs?

Has it accomplished any of the following?
1. Mapped local institutions and formal policy bodies to see where and how rules, laws, and regulations are made that affect our specific goals.
2. Built relationships to gain support of local institutions and formal policy bodies where rules, laws, and regulations are made that affect our goals.
3. Mapped the larger policy arena, including regional and state decision-making bodies, to see where and how policies are made.
4. Built relationships in larger policy arenas.
5. Provided opportunities for community members to participate in mapping, relationship building, and learning advocacy skills.

B. Has the collaboration developed policy strategies?
   1. Has the collaboration identified how its efforts can be sustained through policy and systems change?
   2. Does the collaboration understand barriers to successful implementation of strategies?
   3. Has the collaboration included community members (constituency) in identification, development, and/or refinement of policy strategies?
   4. Has the collaboration provided advocacy opportunities for constituency with decision-making bodies?
C. Has the collaboration been successful at implementing policy and systems change strategies?
   1. How has the collaboration changed rules, regulations, policies, practices, or procedures of local institutions to improve the community?
   2. How has the collaboration influenced policies and legislation to improve child health?
   3. Can the collaboration identify why or why not?

III **The collaboration is sustaining its efforts by spinning off or institutionalizing its effective strategies, activities, or programs.**

A collaboration successful at this sustainability strategy is able to attract resources to continue its successful strategies, but, equally important, sees itself as a catalyst and is proactive in spinning off its effective strategies to local institutions and/or associations.

(Please respond in 1–2 pages. Describe your strengths, challenges, and proposed actions. The Key Questions are to aid you in thinking about this benchmark.)

Key Questions:
A. How has the collaboration been successful in spinning off strategies?
B. How has the collaboration identified potential support?

Has the collaboration considered any of the following prospects? (These are examples for a collaboration focusing on child health.)

Institutions
Local schools
Local government: cities/counties
Community services departments
Parks and recreation

Nonprofits (e.g., community-based organizations, YMCAs, Boys and Girls Clubs, Head Start)
Local Councils (e.g., CPACC—Child Abuse Prevention Council, CCJPC—Child Care Planning Council)
County Children and Families Commission (Prop 10)

Associations
Service clubs—Kiwanis, Rotary, Soroptomists, AAUW
Churches, faith-based organizations, interfaith councils
Neighborhood associations
Chambers of Commerce
Women's networks and business associations

C. How have the collaboration and a mobilized constituency engaged support?

Have they done the following?
1. Identified prospects
2. Built relationships
3. Built case for ongoing support (who we are, what we've done, what we've accomplished, what we need)
4. Gained support

IV The collaboration is sustaining its efforts to improve the community by successfully raising funds and/or proceeding with incorporation to sustain the core functioning of the collaboration.

A collaboration successful at this sustainability strategy wishes to sustain the collaboration itself as an ongoing infrastructure to improve the community. It has attracted resources to sustain this infrastructure or is moving toward incorporation to do the same.

(Please respond in 1–2 pages. Describe your strengths, challenges, and proposed actions. The Key Questions are to aid you in thinking about this benchmark.)

Key Questions:
A. What support has the collaboration already received?
B. How has the collaboration identified additional potential support?

Has the collaboration considered any of the following prospects?
Local government budgets
Local community foundations
Blended local agency funding
State and/or national foundations

    State agencies

    Private donations

    Endowments

    Associations (Chambers of Commerce, interfaith councils)

    Private business

C.   How have the collaboration and a mobilized constituency engaged support?

    Have they done the following?

    1.   Identified potential funders

    2.   Built relationships

    3.   Built case for ongoing support (who we are, what we've done, what we've accomplished, what we need)

    4.   Gained support

D.   Is the collaboration considering incorporation as a sustainability issue? If yes,

    1.   Has the collaboration researched incorporation for feasibility?

    2.   Has the collaboration taken steps to incorporate?

V   The collaboration is making progress in implementing its key strategies (Impact Strategies) to reach its desired outcomes to improve the community.

The successful collaboration not only makes progress on its proposed strategies, but also uses evaluation findings to make revisions when appropriate and necessary. In this way, the collaboration functions as a learning community.

(Please respond in 1–2 pages per Impact Strategy. Describe your strengths, challenges, and proposed actions. The Key Questions are to aid you in thinking about this benchmark.)

Key Questions:

- What are your successes in implementing your strategies?
- What are your challenges?
- What have you learned about these strategies from your evaluation findings?
- What revisions would you like to make on these strategies, based on your evaluation findings?
- What have been your successes in engaging the broader community in your learning community? Does the broader community understand the evaluation findings? Are they involved in

any decisions the collaboration will make based on these findings?
• Have new strategies or opportunities presented themselves that
had not been anticipated? What are they?

Worksheet 9

Coalition Annual Report*

> ***Instructions:*** *Use this sample Coalition Annual Report as a model for communicating with all current and potential coalition members, particular board members, volunteers, contributors and local agency representatives.*

Mission

The Happy Valley Community Coalition is a community-wide alliance committed to improving the quality of life for all those living in Happy Valley.

Goals

- To mobilize and maintain broad-based community development and collaboration problem-solving initiatives around health and human service issues.
- To ensure the availability of, and access to, basic opportunities and services.
- To provide leadership in developing policies, practices, and programs that are effective, responsive, and accountable to those they serve.

Task Force

Coalition Task Forces are formed to address specific needs or issues of concern for Happy Valley residents. During 2000–2001, Task Forces actively addressed health care, transportation, and livable wages.

---

*Hathaway, B. L. (2001). *Lower/Outer Cape Community Coalition annual report 2000–2001*. Eastham, MA: Lower/Outer Cape Community Coalition.

Example 1: Healthy Care Advocacy Task Force

Goal

To increase access to health care, especially for the uninsured, to advocate for local, state, and Federal health policy changes that increase access, and advocate for quality patient care through every stage of medical treatment.

2000–2001 Objectives

✓ To increase Happy Valley residents' usage of the Community Dental Center to 25% of the total participants.
✓ Identify town health needs and resources, and advocate for coordinated responses with Happy Valley health care and other providers.
✓ Implement, track, and evaluate the effectiveness of the coordinated outreach plan for enrollment in MassHealth.
✓ Involve consumers in the evaluation of the Happy Valley Community Dental Center.
✓ Implement a preventive educational dental program in Happy Valley.

Task Force Activities

• Distributed 25,000 pink business cards with phone numbers to call for health insurance enrollment assistance.
• Dental Center evaluation completed by patients.
• Provided informational luncheons for 50 medical office managers on community health center.
• 8 people attended and 3 people testified at the public hearing on May 10 for the Health Now! legislation.
• Participated in the Community Health Access Project (CHAP).

Outcomes

➜ 53.5% of total users of the Dental Care Center are from Happy Valley.
➜ Identified and advocated for health needs of Happy Valley residents.
➜ 690 people enrolled in MassHealth and CMSP.
➜ CHAP efforts brought $1,279,000 in resources to the valley.

Example 2: Business/Nonprofit Partnership

Goal

To increase availability of, and access to, basic opportunities and services for low- and moderate-income wage earners in the Happy Valley.

2000–2001 Objectives

✓ To develop a close working relationship between the business community and the nonprofit sector in Happy Valley, focusing on housing and child care issues.

✓ To provide some employee-related solutions to these issues.

Activities

Two separate groups (Child Care and Housing) were established, which include human service and business members.

Child Care

- A child care committee meets regularly with county child care organizations to coordinate programs and services and exchange information.

Housing

- Encouraged support of local chambers of commerce for local housing proposals.
- A special panel on Happy Valley housing needs and programs was developed to present to the Happy Valley Times editorial board.

Outcomes

➜ The Happy Valley Council on Aging, Happy Valley Chamber of Commerce, and the coalition are developing a pilot shared-housing program, matching elder homeowners and summer employees.

➔ Heightened public awareness of affordable housing needs. *The Happy Valley Times* received an award for their special housing series.

Partners

Happy Valley Children's Place
Happy Valley Chamber of Commerce
Happy Valley Housing Authority
Happy Valley Times
Happy Valley CDC
Happy Valley Community Church

Task Force Worksheet

Task Force's Goal

Year's Objectives

I.
II.
III.
IV.

Activities

→
→
→
→

Outcomes

→
→
→
→

Partners

REFERENCES

Center for Collaborative Planning (2000). *Sustainability Benchmarks*. Sacramento, CA: Author.

Chavis, D., & Florin P. (1990). *Community participation and substance abuse prevention: Rationale, concepts and mechanisms*. County of Santa Clara, CA: Bureau of Drug Abuse Services.

Fawcett, S., Foster, D., & Francisco, V. (1997). Monitoring and evaluation of coalition activities and success. In G. Kaye & W. Wolff (Eds.), *From the ground up: A workbook on coalition building and community development* (pp. 163–185). Amherst, MA: AHEC/Community Partners.

Fetterman, D. (1994). Steps of empowerment evaluation: From California to Cape Town. *Evaluation and Program Planning, 17*(3), 305–313.

Florin, P., & Chavis, D. (1996). *Responsibility charting*. Gaithersburg, MD: Association for the Study and Development of Community.

Francisco, V., & Wolff, T. (1994). Evaluating coalition efforts. *Coalition Building Tip Sheets*. Amherst, MA: AHEC/Community Partners.

Green, L., George, M., Frankish, C., Herbert, C., Bowie, W., & O'Neil, M. (1995). *Study of participatory research in health promotion: Review and recommendations for the development of participatory research in health promotion in Canada*. Ottawa: Royal Society of Canada.

Hathaway, B. L. (1998). *Task force evaluation and resource allocation*. Orleans, MA: Lower/Outer Cape Community Coalition.

Hathaway, B. L. (2001a). Case story #2: Growing a healthy community: A practical guide. *American Journal of Community Psychology, 29*(2), 199–203.

Hathaway, B. L. (2001b). *Lower/Outer Cape Community Coalition annual report (2000–2001)*. Eastham, MA: Lower/Outer Cape Community Coalition.

Hathaway, B. L. (2001c). *Moving from issues to solutions: An evaluation of 13 years of coalition work*. Eastham, MA: Lower/Outer Cape Community Coalition.

Kaye, G. (1993). *Diagnosing your coalition: Risk factors for participation*. Brooklyn, NY: Community Development Associates.

Kaye, G., & Resnick, I. (1994). *Climate diagnostic tool: The six R's of participation*. Brooklyn, NY: Community Development Consultants.

Kaye, G., & Wolff, T. (Eds.) (1997). *From the ground up: A workbook on coalition building and community development*. Amherst, MA: AHEC/Community Partners.

Minkler, M. (2000). Using participatory action research to build healthy communities. *Public Health Reports, 115,* 191–197.

Rosenthal, B. (1997). Multicultural issues in coalitions. In G. Kaye & T. Wolff (Eds.), *From the ground up: A workbook on coalition building and community development* (pp. 51–73). Amherst, MA: AHEC/Community Partners.

Wing, S. (1998). Whose epidemiology, whose health? *International Journal of Health Services, 28,* 241–252.

Wolff, T. (1994). Sustainability of coalitions. *Coalition Building Tip Sheets*. Amherst, MA: AHEC/Community Partners.

CHAPTER 5

Making Sense of Results from Collaboration Evaluations

Vincent T. Francisco, Jerry A. Schultz, and Stephen B. Fawcett

Evaluation of community collaborations has become more and more important, as investments in community collaborations have increased over the past two decades. As the need for evaluation has expanded, tools and resources available for conducting evaluations have become more numerous and accessible. Community collaborations are often engaged in work that changes the context in which whole populations of community members behave. This is a big challenge for the typical evaluator with experience in evaluating individual service programs (e.g., after-school programs for youth), but not in collecting and understanding data about how systems within communities change or in collecting data on behavior change at the level of whole community populations.

With this issue of evaluation need and resources, a similar need has been created for the development of capacity, within community collaborations themselves, to make sense of their data and use those data to improve their collaboration. Often, an evaluator, contracted by a foundation on behalf of a community collaboration or working directly with community collaborations, operates without much contact from the membership. This leaves a big gap in decision making among the leadership within collaborations. That leadership often includes community leaders, policy makers, service agency representatives, and grassroots community members, but they may not have access to resources that help them turn community data into community action. This chapter helps to fill this niche by helping members of community collaborations understand evaluation, make sense of the data they are collecting, and use those data to improve their collaboration.

Evaluation can serve multiple purposes: (1) documenting the implementation of a collaboration; (2) demonstrating effectiveness in accomplishing objectives; (3) providing accountability to grant makers, the community, and other groups interested in the success of the collaboration; (4) increasing community support for collaborations; (5) contributing to the body of scientific knowledge of interventions effective at accomplishing shared goals; and (6) informing policy decisions.

The approaches to evaluation of community collaborations presented here grow out of a number of major movements in research and evaluation practice, including action research (Argyris, Putnam, & Smith, 1990), empowerment evaluation (Fetterman, 1996), and public health and community health promotion (Green & Kreuter, 1991). Excellent information is available on these approaches to evaluation, evaluation tools, and research methodologies (e.g., Centers for Disease Control and Prevention [CDC], 1999; Fawcett et al., 1993, 1995; Linney & Wandersman, 1991), as well as within this volume (see chapter 4) and is not repeated here.

EVALUATION AND PROGRAM PLANNING

Given that all these resources are available, what should a collaboration member, evaluator, technical assistance provider, or grant maker do? What we suggest here is a process of collecting some of the information a collaboration member may already have about their program, extending that information with additional information that might prove useful, and developing a useable evaluation plan. Here are a few reasons to develop such a plan:

- The process of developing a plan helps in deciding what sort of information the members of a community collaboration and their stakeholders really need.
- It helps them clarify reasonable questions, and develop methods and strategies for getting the needed information.
- It helps them come up with a reasonable time line for data collection and providing feedback. The time to begin developing an evaluation plan is when one begins to plan a community collaboration.

Planning and evaluation significantly influence each other. A reasonable process to follow is one suggested by a number of evaluation panels (CDC, 1999; Joint Committee, 1994) and by the evaluation chapters in the Community Tool Box (CTB; *http://ctb.ku.edu/*), and can follow this general outline (adapted from Francisco, Capwell, & Butterfoss, 1999):

1. Clarify your program objectives and goals.
2. Identify your stakeholders and their interests in your program.
3. Develop evaluation questions based on your and your stakeholders' interests.
4. Identify and use evaluation methods that will answer the questions.
5. Set up a time line for evaluation activities and feedback.

There are several additional issues to consider when planning an evaluation of a community collaboration. Important to implementing the evaluation is considering whether there is a need for an external evaluator or whether the evaluation can be conducted with resources internal to a community collaboration. In many cases, collaboration leadership will need an external evaluator. These situations will include a specific requirement stated by the groups funding a program and the need for outside verification that may enhance the credibility of their activities. Outside these conditions, there are many evaluation activities that one can conduct and effectively use to improve a community collaboration.

FRAMING EVALUATION QUESTIONS AND METHODS

Framing evaluation questions is as important as choosing the data collection methods used to answer those questions. There are a number of ways to effectively frame evaluation questions, but, most important, they need to match the framing of the community collaboration. One way to effectively frame a community collaboration is outlined in Figure 5.1.

Framing the Community Collaboration

In this framework, planning a collaboration will be followed by the implementation of the plan, which includes collaboration members developing new programs or interventions targeting youth and adults whose behavior needs to change in order for a shared (perhaps important) outcome to be achieved.

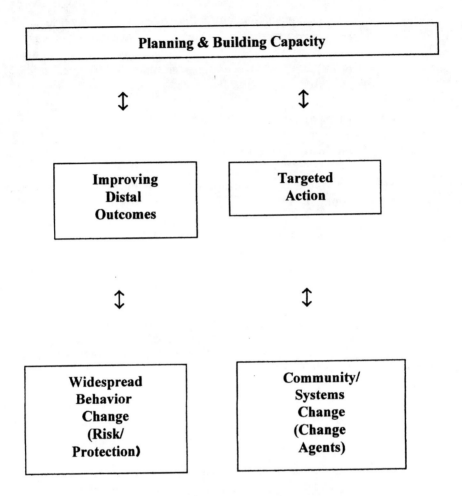

FIGURE 5.1   Framework for community collaboration and improvement.

Additionally, policies will be targeted for implementation or modification, and specific attributes of other programs will be targeted for change. Hopefully, these new or modified programs, policies, and practices (also called community and systems changes) will be implemented in such a way that they will significantly change the behavior of people in the direction of outcomes the community hopes to achieve.

Attributes of these community and systems changes, which will most likely lead to population-level behavior changes, include using effective strategies for behavior change (e.g., alternative activities, modifying the physical design of the environment), depth of penetration into the community-across-community sectors (e.g., faith community, youth-serving agencies, law enforcement) and target populations (e.g., parents, teachers, students), implementing interventions long enough to make a difference, and the sheer number of program and policy changes implemented, so that everyone in the community may benefit from their implementation. Optimistically, these behavior changes, over some period of time, will lead to changes in more distant outcomes that could, for example, include reductions in youth violence or reductions in the rate of deaths from chronic diseases such as diabetes and cardiovascular disease.

Framing Evaluation Questions

Within this framework, a number of relevant questions can be developed, but there is often a long span of time between the development of a community collaboration and the attainment of difficult outcomes. Therefore, it is important to develop some intermediate measures that can help serve to act as indicators of likely success. Five important evaluation questions might be framed to help understand the implementation and accomplishment of this kind of community collaboration:

1. Did the community collaboration facilitate new and modified programs, policies, and practices relevant to the mission of the organization?
2. Is the community satisfied with the collaboration's goals, implementation, and accomplishments?
3. Are the community and systems changes implemented with sufficient duration and intensity of behavior-change strategy, with enough of the target population, and across enough channels of influence in the community, in order to have a significant impact?
4. Did the community collaboration accomplish the goals and objectives it developed?
5. Did the community collaboration bring about changes in more distal markers of community health and development, such as self-reported behavior changes or archival records?

Answering Evaluation Questions

Given these questions, a number of kinds of data can be collected by a community collaboration itself, in order to help understand how the collaboration is unfolding over time, and to help keep the collaboration on track toward success. Questions 1, 3, and 4 can be answered by using logs that record the specific policy changes, program changes, or practice changes that were accomplished through collaboration members meeting with key decision makers who have control over those policies and programs (Francisco, Fawcett, & Paine, 1993). For example, if a group of collaboration members was successful in effecting the acceptance of a law prohibiting the sales of tobacco products to minors, then that law could be considered an accomplishment of the collaboration (at least in part). Such a law would be implemented over a long period of time and, if enforcement were strict, would result in the reduction of tobacco sales to youth.

The use of satisfaction surveys that might focus on one or another of the dimensions of the question might answer question 2. Tools that have been found to be effective in answering this kind of question can be found in the CBT. A survey of goals might be constructed to list the specific objectives for community change and to allow community members to rate each objective by its importance to the mission, and its feasibility. Those objectives that are highly important and highly feasible would be the first that the collaboration might try to accomplish. Those objectives that are highly important and less feasible might become secondary objectives, or might be scheduled for accomplishment over a longer period of time. Those objectives that are rated as less important might be removed from the action plan.

Another kind of satisfaction survey might be useful to collaboration leadership in making sure that all the collaboration members are included in the process of implementation. A satisfaction survey focused on implementation might include questions that ask input on collaboration members' satisfaction with the leadership in general, how the leadership creates opportunities for collaboration members to contribute to success, and how included the collaboration members feel in the decision-making process.

Question 5 would best be answered by the use of self-reported behavior change surveys and other archival records that might be useful in either demonstrating the success of the collaboration in changing the behavior of the community, or in helping to understand how the collaboration might change its objectives to be more successful in accomplishing its goals. There are many self-reported behavior-change surveys that could be useful and more successful in accomplishing its goals. There are many self-reported behavior change surveys that could be useful to community collaborations. Two that are often used in community health and development collaborations are the Behavior Risk Factor Surveillance Survey, and the Youth Risk Behavior Survey, both available from the CDC (*http://www.cdc.gov/*) or from local health departments (in the larger cities). Archival records might include data about the incidence and prevalence of disease (e.g., rates of cardiovascular disease), behavior-related health outcomes (e.g., rates of teen pregnancy, youth tobacco use, or drug use), or other outcomes important to communities (e.g., arrest rates for physical assaults among youth).

MAKING SENSE OF EVALUATION DATA

There are several reasons that a collaboration and its support organizations might consider important in making sense of their data. These reasons parallel the evaluation questions outlined in the previous section. A collaboration could use the process of making sense of their evaluation data to improve its functioning, resulting in greater satisfaction with the collaborative process and in greatly enhanced involvement by community members in the process. It could help to raise community awareness of the issues being addressed by the collaboration, and allow for an improvement in how community members view the collaboration and its success. Additionally, the process of sense making can result in more frequent celebration of accomplishments of the members of the collaboration, which can result in greater numbers of people acting as change agents in the community.

A number of useful resources exist to help make sense of data and to use it to improve functioning and address the outcomes sought by a community collaboration. The most accessible resources might include two areas of the CTB, a Web site that contains many resources relevant to establishing and implementing community collaborations. The first resource is the Evaluation Troubleshooting Guide. This troubleshooting guide is useful, because it contains the questions and advice of many successful evaluators of community collaborations. The first level of the troubleshooting guide contains several issues that collaborations frequently encounter, such as not having brought about many changes in policies or programs in the community, or that community leaders do not value the collaboration and its accomplishments.

Second, it contains questions relating to these issues that can help members of a collaboration (and supportive partners, such as grant makers and evaluators) use their data or collect additional information that might help. The issues might include, "We don't know if our change efforts are using powerful enough strategies for change," or "Our changes don't seem to be reaching our target audience in a way that makes a difference in their lives." Following the Web links associated with these issues will lead to additional tools for successful sense making, and many resources that might not otherwise be available to community groups.

The process of making sense of your data might be seen as incredibly difficult, and the sum total of a graduate school education from a major university, on the one hand, but it is absolutely doable by members of community collaborations with support from resources such as the Evaluation Troubleshooting Guide described above. Also, it could be summarized even more simply by the following procedures.

1. *Describe methods used for analysis and synthesis* (i.e., how did we review the data/information to detect patterns in the evidence?).
2. *State conclusions about what we are seeing.* To do so, characterize the

   • Amount of the intervention/change (e.g., "We haven't brought about enough community and systems change"; "We've seen a decrease in the rate of change")
   • Contribution of community/systems change to addressing the community problem/goal (e.g., "The changes are not there long enough to make a difference")
   • Value of the collaboration and its accomplishments for the key stakeholders (e.g., "The changes don't seem to be important to community members and/or outside experts")
   • Impact of the collaboration (e.g., "We haven't seen any improvement in community-level indicators")
   • Capacity of the community to conduct and use the evaluation (e.g., "We need to evaluate our work, but we don't know how to do it")

3. *Justify any conclusions made from the data* (e.g., "We found that the 155 new or modified programs, policies, and practices facilitated by the collaboration resulted in a reduction in self-reported drug and alcohol use, as reported by the county health department over the past five years").
4. *State the limitations and strengths of the evaluation* (i.e., using standards including utility or usefulness, accuracy or reliability, feasibility or practicality, and propriety or appropriateness (Joint Committee on Standards for Educational Evaluation, 1994).
5. *Ensure protection of the clients and other stakeholders* (Joint Committee, 1994).
6. *Make recommendations about what to celebrate and improve* (i.e., actions to consider taking, based on the evaluation).

It is very important to use the information obtained from the evaluation to celebrate accomplishments and to make adjustments in practice that might lead to enhanced success in accomplishing shared goals. Several things could be done to use the evaluation data to celebrate accomplishments. One important activity that should be conducted by the collaboration is to arrange for group celebrations of community change/improvement. This can take many forms, from printing short articles about successes in a newsletter to holding annual celebrations honoring those people who contributed to the effort (e.g., "champions of change"). Additionally, reports can be written (or visual presentations developed) that communicate data and lessons learned about the collaboration to all key stakeholders, such as grant makers and community leadership. These reports should, at a minimum, provide feedback on what you are seeing (e.g., graphs of data with text describing what the graphs mean), and contain suggestions for how the collaboration can improve over time.

Such reports could form the basis for additional strategic planning, resource development, securing technical assistance and training, and making other kinds of adjustments in practice. This can happen by increasing the amount of the intervention, such as by developing an action plan detailing specific community change objectives, with information about who will accomplish those objectives, what resources are needed, and by when they might be accomplished. Such an action plan might help guide the collaboration members in accomplishing many more policy changes and the development of new programs. The building of new leadership or opportunities for leadership could also increase the effectiveness of the intervention. Our experience has taught us that charismatic leadership is very important to the success of a community collaboration, but that collaboration will be successful for a long period of time only if the charismatic leaders create niches of involvement for all community members to contribute to the success of the collaboration.

Such a report could also lead to enhancing or changing the value of the collaboration and its accomplishments for key stakeholders. One way to do this is to conduct a social marketing effort (e.g., America's Promise for Children), or to provide feedback on the actual effects of the interventions in a form that is accessible to the community (e.g., publishing a community report card).

WORKING TOGETHER TO MAKE A DIFFERENCE IN A COMMUNITY

Evaluation and sense making can be a lot of work, but many collaborations have found that working together with their funding agents and support organizations (such as evaluators and technical assistance providers) can make a big difference in their collective success. In 1999, we published an article (Fawcett et al., 1999) that described what each broad group of stakeholders could do to work together to ensure the success of the community collaboration. In that article, we suggested a "memorandum of collaboration" among the community collaboration, support organizations, and funding agents.

Important to the success of a collaboration are two related activities. One is tracking community data. Collaboration members often are closer to the community members who are doing the work of bringing about community change, and to those people in the community who usually collect outcome data (e.g., police departments, schools). Members of collaborations should work with evaluators and funding agents to broker relationships that can result in access to these data sets. In addition, members of collaborations should help track many of the small wins (small, in that many of them are needed to improve a community) that lead to changes in community outcome data. These small wins (e.g., a new policy allowing youth-serving organizations to freely use school buildings for supervised alternative activities) are often huge accomplishments of collaborations. Support organizations and funding agents should recognize this and facilitate the celebration of these accomplishments.

Valuing community members in this way will not only promote a healthy relationship between these stakeholders, but it can serve the important function of keeping people excited about their work. This kind of positive relationship also helps when it is time to also provide corrective feedback to the collaboration. Framing the feedback as an opportunity to achieve additional success, along with enough support to help the collaboration change, can help ensure success that it might never otherwise achieve. In addition, every coalition and community collaboration goes through lulls in activity and attendance at important events. The celebration of these small wins by members of the collaboration, and by the support organizations, can help recharge the collaboration or launch it into new and exciting directions.

CONCLUDING EXAMPLE

An example follows of an evaluation of The Decade of Hope Coalition, a community collaboration for the prevention of substance abuse on the Jicarilla Apache Reservation, a very rural area in north central New Mexico, and might help illustrate this approach. Challenges the evaluators faced during work on this project are discussed and some lessons learned are presented.

Evaluation Questions and Results

Several evaluation questions were developed in partnership with community members and collaboration implementers. First: Was the community mobilized to address substance abuse? Data were collected, using documentation tools from the CTB, which showed a large number of actions taken to bring about change in the community following the hiring of staff, for the substance abuse coalition, in the spring of 1992. Three staff members accomplished the majority of these actions. One staff member was especially active in facilitating changes herself, rather than mobilizing others to help change the community. But, when staff left the coalition, few additional actions were taken to bring about changes in programs, policies, and practices (as evidenced in the documentation tools). Two additional community mobilizers were hired by the coalition, but without providing an apparent increase in action. Local informants proclaimed the coalition to be effectively inactive.

Using the Evaluation Troubleshooting Guide, we found that more dispersed leadership, beginning with the first mobilizer hired, might have resulted in a less dramatic loss of efficacy for the coalition, and that leadership skill training might have helped. Additionally, perhaps others in the coalition could not take action themselves independent of the community mobilizer. The coalition membership included tribal members who also worked for the tribe. Trying to change the political system would be difficult, because their employment could be adversely affected if the tribal council or their supervisors were targeted for an unpopular change policy or practice change.

What Changes in the Community Resulted from the Coalition?

Data collected with the previously mentioned documentation system suggest that the coalition was very effective in changing programs, policies, and practices relative to its mission of preventing substance abuse. For example, coalition staff succeeded in establishing in-house policies against fighting in local bars. Another important success was the removal of penalties for attendance at health promotion events during working hours, allowing tribal employees to attend workshops on substance abuse awareness sponsored by the coalition, without losing their jobs or any pay for being absent from work.

Many of the programs created during the coalition's most active period have continued, as informally reported by community members. These include programs started as a result of a mini-grants program funded by the coalition.

Examples of mini-grants include an annual ceremony honoring adolescents in the community who demonstrate personal characteristics valued by the community, as well as wilderness experience trips for youth in the custody of the tribe's social services agency.

Do the Changes Reduce Risk for Substance Abuse?

A subanalysis of community changes—by risk factor, strategy, and sector—suggested that actions and accomplishments are not equally distributed across these important domains. Differential feedback on distribution of effects may be important to the success of a coalition. Best practice may involve implementation of policies and programs that affect a wide variety of risk and protective factors, and that use a wide variety of strategies for behavior change in a wide variety of community sectors. If these features do offer the greatest chance for success, then quarterly (or at least annual) reports of this information on effects may provide the initiative leadership and funding agents with data that can be used to make important modifications to implementation of the initiative.

For example, a collaboration's accomplishments may be focused primarily on providing information about risk for substance abuse and what people can do about it. Although this is necessary information, it may not be sufficient to reduce or prevent substance abuse in a community where substance abuse is common. Drift from strategic planning attempts to address this, during the early months of the collaboration, can occur without differential feedback on effectiveness.

Is There a Change in Community-Level Indicators of Substance Abuse?

These data were the most difficult to collect, and the most difficult to interpret. Although the data are incomplete, it was found that a 50% reduction in alcohol-related emergency medical transports occurred during the intervention period of the coalition. As part of the contract negotiations for the evaluation, it was requested that no survey methodology be used, out of respect for their tribal traditions. This limited the range of community-level indicators to what was already collected. Community-level indicators communicate a variety of additional things beyond a summative judgment about impact, and need to be interpreted within the limits of their data collection methodologies.

When we were trying to collect these data, we were often told that the data were not available or would not be made available, because of a lack of trust in how the data would be used. With the local Native American evaluation coordinator as an advocate, we were finally able to get some data. This changed when the evaluator was forced to leave the coalition for personal reasons. The coalition never did replace him, and the impact evaluation never was completed.

In our attempts to follow up with Indian Health Services on the most complete and accurate data (alcohol-related EMS transports), we received data, on two different occasions, that contradicted our earlier data, and that were actually inconsistent. Community-level indicators for substance abuse, and for other health concerns, require careful examination to determine their validity and reliability.

What Critical Events Were Associated With Changes in Rate of Community Change?

Interviews were conducted with key community members and coalition implementers, to help answer this question. Such qualitative data about critical events help give meaning to other more quantitative measures. By integrating qualitative and quantitative data, hypotheses can be generated about key events or factors that may affect the functioning of community collaborations. Critical elements affecting the Decade of Hope coalition include: having paid staff, loss of leadership during the coalition's operation, having a targeted mission, availability of data for monitoring and feedback, and availability of technical assistance on strategic planning.

This process of interviewing collaborations and community members, and the information it provides, is also useful in prompting collaboration participants to reflect on major successes and shortcomings. Focusing on successes allows people, working hard on a potentially intractable problem, an opportunity to celebrate accomplishments. Focusing on shortcomings allows an opportunity to learn about the etiology of mistakes and to make appropriate changes so they do not occur again.

LESSONS LEARNED

This chapter is just an introduction to the use of evaluation in supporting and understanding a community collaboration and in guiding the collaboration through the process of making sense of its data, once collected. Many resources are mentioned in this chapter that are important for members of collaborations to access, review, and use as they implement their collaboration. The most repeated resource in this volume is the CTB. The CTB is a Web site with many links to evaluation tools that can readily be adapted and used within a community collaboration. Mentioned earlier were the troubleshooting guides that summarize issues and questions most frequently encountered by experts and community members with experience implementing community collaborations. Additional resources presented there include two frameworks for program evaluation, which contain a public health approach to evaluating community health collaborations (Chapter 36 Section 1, *http://ctb.ku.edu/tools/EN/section_1338.htm*), and a community development approach to evaluation (Chapter 1 Section 5, *http://ctb.ku.edu/tools/EN/section_1007.htm*).

The foregoing evaluation results, along with our experience with other collaborations, set the stage for a variety of recommendations:

1. *Evaluation should be coupled with appropriate technical assistance.* Work with the Decade of Hope Coalition actually was made more difficult because the funding agency mandated technical assistance packages, both with and without consultation, independent of any demonstrated need from the client—that is, the coalition.

2. *The evaluation should provide early and ongoing feedback.* With the Decade of Hope Coalition, more than a year passed without effective implementation (as evidenced by the lack of community actions and changes). Early feedback can be used to help initiative leadership focus their efforts on taking action in the community, rather than falling into the trap of becoming a support group for members.

3. *The evaluation should occasion celebrations, adjustments, and renewals.* The evaluators should not be seen as watchdogs, or as just providing summative judgments. For example, the critical incident interviews were a productive experience for the Decade of Hope Coalition members, leading to greater enthusiasm on the part of members who took part in the interviews. Additionally, the coalition staff used these data to demonstrate their tremendous activity level to the funding agency and local tribal representatives, which created some buy-in from the tribe. Evaluation should be integrated into the overall process of community development.

4. *Grant makers can and should use contingencies to reinforce progress.* With some funders, grant renewal is not contingent on progress toward fulfilling community change objectives, but is closely tied, instead,

to fiscal accountability. Funders can take an active role in the community development process. Rather than mandate procedures and guidelines for implementation, or fiscal reporting alone, the funders can require progress on accomplishing mutually agreed upon objectives (as demonstrated by evaluation data documenting community changes accomplished by the initiative). In this way, the funders are involved as a catalyst for change and improvement.

5. *Initial community change, measured by an evaluation, may be an important early marker of ultimate outcome.* Changes in impact measures, such as alcohol-related emergency medical transports with the Decade of Hope Coalition, may take a long time to emerge. Additionally, if the mission is affected, impact measures may not be sensitive enough to reliably record those changes. Measures of self-reported behavior change may suffer from similar confounds. A community change of the sort this evaluation gathered may be the most useful interim measure of the success of a collaboration.

6. *Finally, the evaluation should identify particular challenges to long-term success of a collaboration.* With the Decade of Hope Coalition, the evaluation showed a period of quiescence, followed by a period of high activity. This situation should have been addressed by the funders and by coalition leadership. Data collected on community mobilization, and on critical events contributing to community changes, show some factors that could be used to improve functioning and contribute to greater understanding about the community development process in general.

REFERENCES

Argyris, C., Putnam, R., & Smith, D. M. (1990). *Action science.* San Francisco: Jossey-Bass.

Centers for Disease Control and Prevention. (1999). Framework for program evaluation in public health. *Morbidity and Mortality Weekly Report, 48*(RR-11).

Fawcett, S. B., Francisco, V., Paine-Andrews, A., Lewis, R. K., Richter, K. P., Harris, K. J., et al. (1993). *Work group evaluation handbook: Evaluating and supporting community initiatives for health and development.* Lawrence, KS: Work Group on Health Promotion and Community Development, The University of Kansas.

Fawcett, S. B., Francisco, V. T., Paine-Andrews, A., & Schultz, J. A. (1999). Working together for healthier communities: A research-based memorandum of collaboration. *Public Health Reports,* Supplement on Healthy Cities/Healthy Communities.

Fawcett, S. B., Sterling, T. D., Paine-Andrews, A., Harris, K. J., Francisco, V. T., Richter, K. P., et al. (1995). *Evaluating community efforts to prevent cardiovascular diseases.*

Atlanta, GA: Centers for Disease Control and Prevention, National Center for Chronic Disease Prevention and Health Promotion.

Fetterman, D. M. (1996). Empowerment evaluation: An introduction to theory and practice. In D. M. Fetterman, S. J. Kaftarian, & A. Wandersman (Eds.), *Empowerment evaluation: Knowledge and tools for self-assessment and accountability* (pp. 3–46). Thousand Oaks, CA: Sage.

Francisco, V. T., Capwell, E., & Butterfoss, F. D. (2000). Getting off to a good start with your evaluation. *Journal of Health Promotion Practice, 1*(2), 126–131.

Francisco, V. T., Fawcett, S. B., & Paine, A. L. (1993). A method for monitoring and evaluating community coalitions. *Health Education Research: Theory and Practice, 8*(3), 403–416.

Green, L. W., & Kreuter, M. W. (1991). *Health promotion planning* (2nd ed.). Mountain View, CA: Mayfield.

Joint Committee on Standards for Educational Evaluation. (1994). The program evaluation standards. *Evaluation Practice, 15,* 334–336.

Linney, J. A., & Wandersman, A. (1991). *Prevention Plus III: A Four-Step Guide to Useful Program Assessment.* Rockville, MD: U.S. Department of Health and Human Services.

CHAPTER **6**

Evaluating Collaborations in Youth Violence Prevention

Nancy G. Guerra

Community efforts to understand and prevent youth violence take on many forms: collaborations, coalitions, prevention networks, community action networks, initiatives, task forces, partnerships, and so on. They also take on many tasks. Given the sheer number of these collaborative endeavors in the United States in recent years, it is not surprising to find considerable variation in the set of tasks they take on. In some cases, their main focus is strategic planning, whether as an ongoing process or to produce a comprehensive document (i.e., a community strategic plan for youth violence prevention). In other cases, their mandate is to develop a program or set of programs to be implemented following the planning phase. In still other cases, their activities are directed toward involving the entire community in an ongoing, synergistic violence prevention effort that is woven into the local ecology.

Given the time and dollars invested in building community youth violence prevention collaborations over the last several decades, there is also a keen awareness of the need to demonstrate their impact. The focus on impact is particularly critical in the area of youth violence prevention, because of the urgency of the problem and the finite (and often limited) resources available to address it. This need has resulted in a heightened sensitivity to the importance of evaluation in the collaborative process. Still, there is much variation in both the type and extent of evaluation being conducted at the local level.

In practice, integrating evaluation into the ongoing work of youth violence prevention collaborations poses several challenges.

The purpose of this chapter is to explore these challenges and suggest ways they may be overcome. A diverse literature is examined, including case studies of related community efforts. The author also draws on personal experience providing technical assistance to youth violence prevention strategic planning projects funded by the John S. and James. L. Knight Foundation. Five major evaluation challenges faced by youth violence prevention collaborations are discussed:

- Determining the scope of the evaluation
- Confronting difficulties inherent in evaluating complex and flexible activities
- Differentiating information-gathering and needs assessment from evaluation
- Identifying measures, collecting assessments, and presenting data
- Selecting an evaluator

In addition to a discussion of these challenges, there is a suggested framework for evaluation that emphasizes *monitoring, learning, and impact*. That framework differentiates between evaluating activities and functions of the collaboration per se and evaluating the implementation and impact of selected youth violence prevention and intervention programs. The discussion covers how this framework can be helpful in addressing each of the challenges presented, and concludes with some general recommendations.

THE KNIGHT FOUNDATION INITIATIVE TO PROMOTE YOUTH DEVELOPMENT AND PREVENT YOUTH VIOLENCE

In 1995, the trustees of the John S. and James L. Knight Foundation approved embarking on a comprehensive Initiative to Promote Youth Development and Prevent Youth Violence. Funds from this initiative were made available in all 26 communities served by Knight Foundation, for either a planning or an implementation project. Planning grants were awarded to 13 communities: Biloxi, MS; Boulder, CO; Bradenton, FL; Charlotte, NC; Columbia, SC; Columbus, GA; Detroit, MI; Grand Forks, ND; Lexington, KY; Macon, GA; Milledgeville, GA; Myrtle Beach, SC; and St. Paul, MN. These 1-year grants supported development of a comprehensive strategic plan to address youth violence, and required a collaboration and participatory process in the development and approval of this plan. Knight Foundation would then consider some of the programmatic recommendations for a possible implementation grant, although funding for these implementation projects was allocated through a separate process and was not automatic.

Planning grantees were required to conduct a local evaluation. In addition, the foundation commissioned a two-part external evaluation of the planning grants. The first part of the evaluation was an evaluability assessment, designed to assess progress by the 13 projects toward their goals and to assess difficulties encountered along the way, as well as to determine what additional evaluation activities would be appropriate (Backer, 2000). The results of the evaluability assessment included a plan for a modest cross-site evaluation that focused on three objectives: (1) assessing the impact and postplanning grant status of the 13 collaborations created for these planning projects; (2) exploring what uses had been made of the strategic plans that each project created; and (3) determining what happened to planning project staff after the end of the planning period, including their longer-term commitments to addressing youth violence in their communities.

CHALLENGES TO EVALUATION

The Knight Foundation planning grants were intended to build a collaboration structure that would produce a comprehensive community strategic plan for youth violence prevention. The defined and circumscribed nature of the tasks rendered evaluation more manageable. Still, the grantees struggled with many of the same evaluation concerns faced by collaborations with a broader mandate. These challenges are also similar to challenges faced by any type of collaboration focused on health promotion or prevention of social problems. The five challenges to be discussed here are:

- determining the scope of the evaluation
- confronting difficulties inherent in evaluating complex and flexible activities
- differentiating information-gathering and needs assessment from evaluation
- identifying measures, collecting assessments, and presenting data
- selecting an evaluator

The following discussions also include recommendations for how evaluators and community organizations may deal better with these five challenges.

Determining the Scope of the Evaluation

Just as there are many possible tasks for collaborations to take on, there are also many types and levels of possible evaluation. Often, the scope of the evaluation is fixed by the funding entity, and can range from almost nothing (except perhaps a brief report), to a "learning lab" approach, to a required comprehensive process and outcome evaluation. Collaborations that are locally funded typically have fewer evaluation mandates than those that are funded by foundation, state, or federal sources. When evaluations are required, their emphasis often depends on the funding agency's approach to evaluation, as well as on the specific requirements of the initiative.

The statewide Colorado Healthy Communities Initiative, funded by the Colorado Trust from 1992 to 1998, is an example of a learning approach to evaluation, which characterizes the evaluation strategy typically used by the Colorado Trust. In this initiative, a total of 28 communities developed their vision of a healthy community and created strategic plans to move toward their goals. The Colorado Trust (1998) also invested in an evaluation of this multiyear, multisite process, which focused primarily on documenting "lessons learned." Many of those lessons learned (e.g., collaboration leaders are essential to a successful project, offering implementation funding invariably affects the planning process, and significant change takes time) were then used to guide similar collaboration efforts, including a 26-community youth violence prevention initiative.

Alternatively, when a major focus of the collaboration process is to develop an implementation project in a community, the scope of the evaluation may focus on the success of the implementation project in impacting targeted outcomes. For example, during the mid-1990s, the National Funding Collaboration on Violence Prevention (NFCVP) used this type of approach. NFCVP was founded in 1995 as a type of collaboration across funding sources for community-based violence prevention. Nearly 30 funding sources (including federal agencies and foundations) were involved. With these funds, proposals were solicited from local community foundations to form violence prevention collaborations to address many different types of community violence.

The thinking behind this approach was that violence prevention required a comprehensive strategy that must be implemented by a collaboration of organizations and citizens working together. A major task of the collaboration was to design and implement comprehensive strategies that included specific programs. Eleven local collaborations across the United States participated in planning and implementing community-based violence prevention projects. Evaluation was not a part of the planning process, but was seen as a component of implementation. Indeed, a final planning activity was to select a local evaluator and develop an evaluation plan for the implementation phase of the initiative (COSMOS, 1997).

In some cases, the type and extent of evaluation are determined by state mandate. For example, the evaluation of the Rhode Island Substance Abuse Prevention Act, as reported by Florin, Mitchell, and Stevenson (1993), involved a mandate by the state legislature to conduct a process and implementation evaluation. This was accomplished via a contract to the Community Research and Services Team. The evaluation team worked with 35 community coalitions to assess progress with initial coalition-building tasks, quality of the strategic plans, implementation of activities designed to change individuals and communities and, ultimately, changes in substance-use behavior.

The Knight Foundation planning grants were required to conduct a local evaluation and to participate in a cross-site evaluation commissioned by the foundation. Projects were given considerable leeway in structuring the local evaluation. They were asked to emphasize documentation of activities and lessons learned. The cross-site evaluation provided an opportunity to collect additional information about the community strategic plan. Indicators of impact of the strategic plan included overall quality of the document, as rated by independent consultants; number of agencies using the strategic plan, after the planning process had been completed and at follow-up; and amount of additional monies for youth violence prevention generated as a direct result of the collaboration's activities.

Even when evaluation guidelines are provided by a funding agency, collaborations often have trouble when it comes to the details of the evaluation. Requiring a process or outcome evaluation may provide some guidance regarding what is expected, but there is still much to be decided. This is exacerbated by the many difficulties inherent in evaluating this type of effort.

Confronting Difficulties Inherent in Evaluating Complex and Flexible Activities

The complexity and flexibility of collaborations make them difficult to evaluate. Rather than a circumscribed set of events with a beginning, middle, and end, and with specified and measurable activities, collaborations involve multiple players, multiple systems, and a changing series of activities. This is further complicated because no two collaborations unfold in quite the same fashion, making comparative studies even more problematic. For this reason, most evaluations of violence prevention collaborations provide a compilation of case studies, with cross-site analyses aimed at identifying similar experiences and their impact (Backer, 2001; COSMOS, 1997).

In describing the challenges of studying comprehensive collaboration services, Knapp (1995) identifies a number of challenges that are relevant for evaluating community violence prevention collaborations. These include:

- Engaging divergent participants' perspectives
- Characterizing and measuring the elusive independent variable
- Locating and measuring the bottom line
- Attributing results to influences.

By definition, collaborations involve a diverse group of participants and stakeholders. For example, most youth violence prevention collaborations typically are comprised of representatives from the justice system, youth-service agencies, schools, faith community, health services, child protective services, city/county government, parents, youth, and others. Adequately representing each of these perspectives in an evaluation strategy is not an easy task. In addition, participants often differ significantly in their support of evaluation, in general, and in their understanding of what it takes to conduct an adequate evaluation.

As Knapp (1995) notes, characterizing the independent variable—those programmatic activities presumed to be responsible for individual or systemic change—is complex. In more traditional intervention research, the independent variable, typically equivalent to the treatment, is clearly specified, monitored, and delivered systematically. For youth violence prevention collaborations, the treatment can range from a minimal effort to coordinate services, to an intensive, highly integrated network of services that attempts to influence a range of individual and environmental risk factors for violence. Further, because collaboration activities involve multiple players in diverse settings, whose activities often change over time, precisely what has occurred is often difficult to document.

Just as defining the specific collaboration activities believed to influence desired outcomes poses distinct challenges, defining the desired outcomes, or the bottom line, may be equally elusive. Any number of plausible outcomes of youth violence prevention collaborations can be identified. Were new programs developed? Were additional funds for youth violence prevention brought into the community? Were positive community changes observed? Were members satisfied with the collaboration? Were community members satisfied? Was the strategic plan of high quality? Was it well received? Were changes in collaboration practices identified? Were changes in individual and/or community-level indicators of youth violence noted?

In practice, both funders and collaboration members are often eager to see their efforts result in reductions in levels of youth homicide and other types of serious youth violence. These concerns tend to grow exponentially as the work of the collaboration enters the political arena. Most politicians want to be associated with projects that work, meaning that they work to reduce violence, not work to get people to coordinate their services or like each other more. Thus, there is often spoken or unspoken pressure to achieve reductions in youth violence.

Even if changes in outcomes most linked to youth violence prevention are noted, how can collaborations determine whether these changes were brought about by their activities? Many factors contribute to youth violence at the individual, social contextual, and environmental levels (Tolan & Guerra, 1994). Youth violence prevention collaborations, including those that provide for a range of integrated prevention services, are still but one set of forces in a community. In practice, the journey from collaboration planning to reducing youth violence probably is one of a thousand steps that may take years to achieve. The collaboration's activities may also be a necessary but not sufficient component of an even broader response to youth violence.

Indeed, evaluations rarely document other equally plausible forces and their impact. This is particularly problematic in large communities or cities where the collaboration group may be but one of many strategies or activities focused on youth violence prevention. The collaboration may exist, in fact, because of a surge in funding for violence prevention, often in response to increased public awareness and concern after a killing or notoriously violent event. In some cases, there may also be more than one collaboration group. For example, one of the grants funded by the Knight Foundation went to a city youth violence prevention task force. However, within a few months (and using a different funding source), the school district linked up with a local hospital to form a different youth violence prevention planning group, with both groups operating in tandem for quite a while.

In addition to broad challenges, such as defining the scope of the evaluation and trying to demonstrate outcomes linked to a complex and flexible set of activities, youth violence prevention collaborations also face specific challenges related to the pragmatic aspects of their evaluation. These include challenges related to decisions about types and function of data to be collected, selection of assessments, and selection of an evaluator.

Differentiating Information-Gathering and Needs Assessment From Evaluation

Commonly, violence prevention coalitions (as well as substance prevention and other similar efforts) begin the collaboration process by focusing on gathering community indicators. These indicators are used to determine the extent of the local problem; comparison to county, state, and/or national data; services available; gaps in services; associated risk factors; and other related information. Violence prevention collaborations typically gather data on indicators such as juvenile arrests by type of crime, child welfare data, and gang activity by location (e.g., census tracts). They also frequently compile rosters of violence prevention programs available and identify areas of most need (e.g., programs for very young children, programs in certain communities).

This type of information-gathering serves many purposes, including getting people past denial of the problem, providing a common information base, providing a model for collaboration, providing an empirically based needs assessment, and providing a basis for monitoring and evaluating change (Gabriel, 1997). However, in and of itself, providing a process or outcome assessment of the violence prevention collaboration is not sufficient, although these data may be used as baseline data for outcome assessment. Otherwise put, if the collaboration goes no further than collecting initial information on community indicators, it will have done little in the way of evaluation of the collaboration or its products.

This is not to say that the evaluator or evaluation team cannot be helpful in collecting these data. In fact, some models for evaluating community initiatives stress the importance of involving the evaluation team in all phases of coalition building. Consider empowerment evaluation, which has had a significant influence on the field (Fawcett et al., 1996). According to this framework, the evaluator works as part of a support team that is involved in all phases of the planning process, including collecting epidemiological data on incidence and prevalence of identified problems and assessing available resources. Still, within an empowerment framework, this type of data collection is part of a larger evaluation process, rather than a stand-alone activity.

Identifying Measures, Collecting Assessments, and Presenting Data

Access to instruments or assessments for gauging progress can greatly facilitate the evaluation process. These include simple logs to record activities (e.g., persons contacted, meetings, public forums, attendees), interview protocols for collecting process data, measures of community indicators, and individual assessments of risk/protective factors and behaviors linked to violence and other associated outcomes.

However, collaborations often do not know where to find these instruments. They often spend a fair amount of time developing forms, searching for assessments, and writing their own questionnaires. There are few resources that provide a compendium of needed measures for violence prevention collaborations or that help collaborations explore how to collect data and present information. Collaborations often rely on technical assistance providers or consultants to access this information for them.

The author's own experience with the Knight Foundation grantees involved searching various databases, Web sites, and reference listings for useful books or articles, and identifying only a few that were really helpful to grantees. An article by Francisco, Paine, and Fawcett (1993), "A Methodology for Monitoring and Evaluating Community Health Coalitions," was found to be particularly helpful by the projects.

Several of the Knight Foundation planning grantees decided to do community surveys to gather information on an assortment of indicators, to measure either current issues prior to planning or how communities were different after planning: citizen perceptions of youth violence and youth needs, beliefs about the causes of violence, familiarity with services available, perceptions of services needed, fear of crime, family supports, and changes in the community. To measure these (or whatever combination they chose) indicators, they often set about writing a list of questions for a community survey.

In one instance, the collaboration had developed a 122-item survey and planned to do a random mailing to 1,000 households. However, they were quickly overwhelmed by the sheer size of the survey and extent of the data that might confront them (assuming a decent response rate). When the consultants suggested to them that their survey was too long and too complicated for their purposes, they were actually greatly relieved. They were informed that focus groups would be a more manageable activity, if conducted at various stages of the planning process, and could serve as a source of both process and outcome information. Fortunately, their foray into survey research was short-lived.

Selecting an Evaluator

Ideally, an evaluator should be able to help collaborations navigate the complexities of evaluation, assist with multiple decisions along the way, and minimize the evaluation burden. However, many collaborations have trouble selecting an evaluator, for several reasons. In settings where evaluation is mostly left to the collaboration, there are often limited funds available. Given this restriction, members may have difficulty deciding whether to hire an outside consultant or to conduct the evaluation internally (e.g., by the coordinator or a member of the collaboration). Even when funds are available to hire an external evaluator, there may be a shortage of local consultants with expertise in evaluation of collaborations, and even fewer consultants who are also knowledgeable about youth violence prevention.

Members of the collaboration also may not have the knowledge and/or leeway to select an evaluator whose approach is best suited to the group's needs. Moreover, they may not have the experience to adequately assess the needs of the collaboration and how they will use information gathered. This is particularly problematic, given that there are many different models and theories of evaluation, each suggesting a different course of action and type of evaluator.

In many cases, evaluation is seen as an integral part of the collaboration process. Indeed, several popular models or typologies of evaluation emphasize the interconnectedness of planning and evaluation. These include utilization-focused evaluation, with its emphasis on intended use by intended users (Patton, 1978); developmental evaluation, with its role in program development (Patton, 1994); and empowerment evaluation, designed to promote participation in the evaluation process and use of results (Fawcett et al., 1996). When the evaluator is part of the project team, using evaluation to enhance the work of the collaboration is also important.

Indeed, most types of participatory evaluations are based on the notion of a continuous feedback loop, whereby data and other information are fed back to members of the collaboration on a regular basis, so that midcourse successes and needed corrections can be identified. In some cases, the evaluation is mostly an ongoing process of communication that can last for several years. As Patton (1994) notes in describing evaluation as a long-term partnership, "Developmental programming calls for developmental evaluation in which the evaluator becomes part of the design team helping to monitor what's happening, both process and outcomes, in an evolving, rapidly changing environment of constant feedback and change" (p. 313).

Of course, this type of confluent process requires a high level of commitment to the evaluation process, including a mechanism for regular feedback from the local evaluator. Some evaluation models emphasize the role of the evaluator in program development and decision making about best practices. For violence prevention collaborations, this would require that the evaluator be skilled in program evaluation and have up-to-date knowledge of the violence prevention literature.

In practice, most evaluators are not experts in youth violence prevention, but tend to be generalists with knowledge of evaluation and research design. Further, their time commitments often are limited. Most of the changes that occur over the course of a collaboration's work come from within, that is, from observations and discussions among members. In some cases, the members of the collaboration may even have difficulty communicating effectively with the evaluator, or vice versa.

One case in particular comes to mind, from the Knight Foundation projects. A planning collaboration had been struggling to find an identity and direction, in part, because of changes in staffing, the addition of new members, and changes in the local funding picture. All in all, the end result was a rather shaky level of self-confidence in their collective capabilities. In an attempt to rekindle their sense of direction, the collaboration hired a new evaluation consultant from the local university and made the evaluator part of the project team. At one meeting, the consultant presented an elaborate set of logic models with arrows going in almost every direction. Everyone from the collaboration was rather quiet, nodding occasionally in seeming approval. After the meeting, during a more informal lunch, one of the members was asked whether she was satisfied with the evaluation plan. She waited for a moment without answering, until told that others had found it almost impossible to follow what was presented, to which she replied, "Oh, thank goodness, I thought that I just didn't understand research."

Work with other Knight Foundation projects revealed that most groups had a difficult time finding evaluators, and generally chose someone they knew and liked, regardless of the match with project needs. In general, partnerships with consultants worked better than partnerships with university faculty who had regular academic commitments. This may have been because the academic evaluators chosen were not trained in community psychology or a related field and were more aligned with traditional experimental research methods. Such training may be more appropriate for evaluating implementation projects (or the implementation phase of planning projects). For example, the cross-site evaluation of the local projects funded by the NFCVP reported that collaborations recruited an "excellent cadre of mainly academically-based evaluators. The local evaluation plans were, for the most part, realistic and responsive to the conditions imposed by the local collaborations" (COSMOS, 1997, p. 30).

FRAMEWORK FOR EVALUATING COMMUNITY YOUTH VIOLENCE PREVENTION COLLABORATIONS

The many challenges youth violence prevention collaborations face in designing and conducting evaluations suggest a need to set out guidelines that allow us to address some of these challenges and to simplify the evaluation process. What follows is a proposed framework that emphasizes monitoring, learning, and impact, and differentiates between the planning and action functions of community youth violence prevention collaborations. It also allows for specification of data to be collected, including, for example, who should collect it and the type of measure. Clear specification of the scope of the evaluation and related tasks should also provide needed guidance in selecting the most appropriate evaluator.

The scope of any evaluation will depend to a great extent on the specific goals of the collaboration. These goals can be divided into two primary categories: (a) collaboration activities directed toward planning a specific violence prevention activity, set of activities, or strategic community response (planning phase), and (b) implementation of selected violence prevention programs or responses that are directly aimed at preventing or reducing youth violence (implementation phase). Collaborations may engage in planning only, implementation only, or both planning and implementation. They may also decide to focus their evaluation on only one particular phase, as illustrated by the emphasis on evaluation of implementation for projects funded by the NFCVP.

In addition, evaluations can serve multiple purposes. Three common purposes are monitoring, learning, and impact assessment. These represent increasingly more labor-intensive and time-consuming tasks. In other words, monitoring primarily requires record keeping of activities, events, and participation. Learning requires feedback about processes, including what is working well, what is not working well, possible changes, and how future endeavors might be done differently. This type of feedback tends to be both informal (e.g., discussions among collaboration members) and formal (e.g., consumer satisfaction surveys, interviews, focus groups). Finally, a focus on impact requires specification of desired goals and how they will be achieved and measured. An important component of an impact evaluation involves linking these goals with activities; thus, impact evaluations require adequate attention to monitoring and learning, as well. Table 6.1 provides examples of the type of information youth violence prevention collaborations might collect to address evaluation goals of monitoring, learning, and impact for both the planning phase and the implementation phase.

How might collaborations decide on a focus for their evaluation? First, this depends on whether they are involved in planning or some combination of planning and implementation. Second, they must identify which component is most important to evaluate and must specify the purpose of the evaluation (which may be determined a priori by the funding agency). Let us now turn

TABLE 6.1 Overview of Framework for Evaluating Youth Violence Prevention Collaborations

Phase	Monitoring	Learning	Impact
Planning Collaboration activities directed toward planning a specific violence prevention activity, set of activities, or strategic community response	• Members recruited • Number of youth recruited • Diversity of membership • Number of meetings • Number of forums • Attendance at meetings and forums • Number and type of youth-led activities • List of agencies contacted for needs assessment	• What is working well • How to increase attendance • How to engage youth • How to best collect data on youth violence • How to engage community members • How to involve hard-to-reach constituents	• Consensus on vision • Increased collaboration among members in community • Increased sensitivity to diverse needs • Additional monies for programs • Quality of strategic plan • Agencies using strategic plan • Policy changes
Implementation Implementation of selected violence prevention programs or responses that are directly aimed at reducing youth violence	• Number of youth and families served • Quality of implementation • Fidelity of implementation • Adaptations and changes • Monies spent per youth/family	• What factors determine whether youth and families attend • Do clients represent diversity in the community; if not, how can others be reached • What is working well and how can services be improved • How can services be better linked together	• Client improvement on proposed mediators (or proximal outcomes) • Family or others' improvement on proposed mediators • Individual differences on violence or related behaviors • Moderators of impact (e.g., for whom did the program work best) • Changes in community indicators

to a discussion of how this framework can be used to describe the evaluation activities carried out by the Knight-funded planning projects.

The Knight Foundation was interested in the monitoring, learning, and impact of the planning phase. The monitoring tasks (e.g., documenting participation, diversity, and community engagement) were left to the local evaluator. The learning tasks were included in the local evaluation and the cross-site assessment. The local evaluation information was integrated into a brief lessons-learned document, focused on how to enhance the work of the local collaborations (Guerra, 1998). The cross-site external evaluation was oriented toward impact assessment, with a particular focus on the quality and use of the community strategic plan (Backer, 2001).

For example, there was wide variation in how strategic plans were formatted and disseminated to their communities. Some communities produced short documents with no artwork, which were copied; other communities produced sophisticated print publications in several colors, with advanced graphics and pictures. In terms of dissemination, one community went door-to-door distributing its plan, another community printed 50,000 copies and sent it home with every school child in the community, and another project disseminated its plan on-line. Clearly, some strategic plans were better than others, both in terms of quality of the document and extent of its dissemination.

Although not directly linked to the quality of the strategic plan, the external evaluation noted several funded and unfunded spin-off projects that were clearly related to the work of the collaborations. These included a youth assistance program funded by the local Kiwanis Club, an increase in funding for school security from the local school district, a $1 million federal grant for early-prevention programming, and various grant submissions to local, state, and federal agencies. Other types of systems-change activities were also noted, including a regular community forum that provides opportunities for citizens to speak out; the addition of a mentoring component to an ongoing program, a change in funding priorities for a local foundation, to include an emphasis on youth violence prevention; and a new dialogue among local grantmakers, focused on how to enhance funding and programs for youth violence prevention.

Evaluation of the implementation phase of collaboration work is more complex. If collaborations are implementing one or more specific youth violence prevention programs, they need to evaluate each program separately. This raises a number of issues related to the difficulty in evaluating prevention and intervention programs in the field, which are particularly critical when trying to assess outcomes and link them to programming. In terms of monitoring, most programs keep records of number of clients served and service hours per client or family.

Using this information, calculating cost per client is also relatively easy. However, issues such as quality of implementation and implementation fidelity are often harder to document. Although some interventions are manualized and follow a detailed protocol, many programs involved services such as counseling and supervision, which may vary greatly from client to client and program to program. Learning about how to enhance the program often occurs informally via discussions among program staff. However, to the extent that this results in ongoing programmatic changes to enhance services, it renders evaluation of outcomes even more problematic.

As mentioned previously, most collaborations and agencies have a difficult time selecting appropriate indicators of impact and assessments to measure them. Evaluation consultants should be able to help with this task, and often do. However, all too frequently, consultants spend the bulk of their time helping agencies develop complex logic models that result in a type of evaluation paralysis. This is because evaluation based on these logic models require the assessment of multiple proximal outcomes (e.g., attitude change, family functioning) and distal outcomes (e.g., violence), and include a complex assessment and data analyses plan that could determine whether change in distal outcomes is indeed mediated by changes in proximal outcomes (according to the program's theory of change). Even in the most sophisticated prevention research studies, these relations are difficult to demonstrate. Certainly, such designs are beyond the capacity and funding allocation for most projects implemented by collaborations. Rather than try to measure every possible outcome, projects would do well to select realistic (and easily measurable) indicators.

In addition to a focus on individual program outcomes, collaborations may also want to determine the synergy or collective impact of multiple programs, as is typically the case with violence prevention collaborations that are ongoing and responsible for creating and sustaining a range of programs. Indeed, when planning projects make the transition to implementation projects, they often include a range of prevention and intervention activities. For example, in the case of the NFCVP, prevention activities included media campaigns, enhanced police–community relations, leadership development, weapons abatement, comprehensive truancy prevention, multiparty gang mediation, housing rehabilitation, economic development, and employment.

Other collaborations may be less oriented toward planning and more focused on enhancing community-based services. One example of such an ongoing effort is the Violence Prevention Coalition of Greater Los Angeles, a public–private partnership founded in 1991, with more than 800 members. The coalition receives funds from various sources and engages in numerous activities, including public awareness campaigns, engaging youth in dialogue about violence, providing challenge grants to local programs, and hosting a biennial violence prevention conference (for more information, see Little Hoover Commission, 2001). Frequently, indicators do not show corresponding changes, or get worse. Even when youth violence decreases, demonstrating (to any reasonable level of confidence) that these changes are linked outcomes is virtually impossible, because these multiprogram efforts typically focus on changes in community indicators of violence.

GENERAL RECOMMENDATIONS

Given the complexities in evaluating the work of youth violence prevention collaborations, particularly as related to changes in youth violence, what can a collaboration do to assess its effectiveness? Clearly, this decision depends on local capacity, interests, needs, and priorities, as well as on requirements from the funding agency. Based on experience working with such collaborations, the following recommendations are offered:

- *Be certain about the evaluation requirements for your funding agency (or oversight agency).* In many cases, collaborations are asked to write an evaluation plan, but guidelines from the funding agency are vague and unspecified.
- *Be careful to select an evaluator who shares your ideas about the scope of the evaluation and the role of the evaluator.* Allow time for discussions about what type of evaluation is desired and what type of evaluator is best (e.g., someone who is very engaged from the start or someone who does a postplanning assessment only).
- *Be realistic about what you can assess and what you will learn from that assessment.* There is certainly nothing wrong with doing a good job of monitoring progress for planning or implementation projects, if that is all that is feasible. Problems typically arise when collaborations try to do more than they are capable of doing (given funding, availability of consultants, and types of activities).
- *Understand that youth violence has many causes and that a single program or project is unlikely to have a sizable impact.* Educating funders and policy makers about the difficulty in preventing youth violence is also important, in order for them to have reasonable expectations about program outcomes.
- *Embrace qualitative methods that include feedback and suggestions from all parties involved.* Given the difficulty in conducting scientifi-

cally rigorous evaluations of youth violence prevention and intervention programs, more attention should be paid to listening to the voices of those who are served and those who provide services. In addition to providing information about how to better serve youth and families, participants are the best judges of whether programs are meeting their needs and helping them stay away from violence.

REFERENCES

Backer, T. E. (2000). *Final report: Knight Youth Violence Prevention Initiative: Planning grant evaluability assessment.* Encino, CA: Human Interaction Research Institute.

Backer, T. E. (2001). *Cross-site evaluation for the planning phase of Knight Foundation's Initiative to Promote Youth Development and Prevent Youth Violence.* Encino, CA: Human Interaction Research Institute.

The Colorado Trust (1998). *Lessons from the field: The Colorado Healthy Communities Initiative.* Denver: Author.

COSMOS Corporation (1997). *Communities preventing violence: A cross-site report on the planning period of local violence prevention collaborations.* Washington, DC: Author.

Fawcett, D., et al. (1996). Empowering community health initiatives through evaluation. In D. M. Fetterman, S. J. Kaftarian, & A. Wandersman (Eds.), *Empowerment evaluation: Knowledge and tools for self assessment and accountability* (pp. 165–194). Thousand Oaks, CA: Sage.

Florin, P., Mitchell, R., & Stevenson, J. (1993). Identifying training and technical assistance needs in community coalitions: A developmental approach. *Health Education Research, 8,* 417–432.

Francisco, V. T., Paine, A. L., & Fawcett, S. B. (1993). A methodology for monitoring and evaluating community health coalitions. *Health Education Research, 8,* 403–416.

Gabriel, R. M. (1997). Community indicators of substance abuse: Empowering coalition planning and evaluation. *Evaluation and Program Planning, 20,* 335–343.

Guerra, N. G. (1998). *"Lessons learned" from the Knight Foundation Planning Grants.* Report submitted to the John S. and James L. Knight Foundation, Miami.

Knapp, M. S. (1995). How shall we study comprehensive, collaboration services for children and families? *Educational Researcher, 24,* 5–16.

Little Hoover Commission (2001). *Never too early, never too late to prevent youth crime and violence.* Sacramento, CA: Author.

Patton, M. Q. (1978). *Utilization-focused evaluation.* Beverly Hills, CA: Sage.

Patton, M. Q. (1994). Developmental evaluation. *Evaluation Practice, 15,* 311–319.

Tolan, P. H., & Guerra, N. G. (1994). *What works in preventing youth violence.* Boulder, CO: Center for the Study and Prevention of Violence.

Commentary

John Bare

Funders and community collaborations are continually searching for meaningful ways to work together. It is often a difficult match to make. Aside from the fact that funders have money to give away and community collaborations need it, their interests may not be mutual.

Funders with clear missions look for investments that will advance their strategic objectives. In today's evaluation parlance, this is about outcomes. Increasingly, foundation boards want to sharpen the focus of their grant making in order to heighten the impact. Board and staff may adopt outcome indicators for which the foundation will hold itself accountable. Yet funders, unless they are operating foundations, need strong nonprofit partners to implement activities designed to produce these outcomes. This positions funders as wholesalers in the business of social change, with community collaborations functioning as retailers.

Community collaborations, of course, must respond to many needs other than those of a funder. Partners in the collaboration have unique needs. Community stakeholders may be impatient for results. Collaborations require infusions of energy that refresh and sustain the effort. The authors in this volume have described in detail the many pressures that affect evaluations of community collaborations. The tug of these disparate forces, each with its own reporting requirements, can pull community collaborations in many different directions. A community collaboration might collapse under this weight. Given the respective interests of funders and community collaborations, finding the right match between funders and community collaborations requires careful preparation, to identify the point at which the respective missions overlap—or, in some cases, to figure out that the overlap is either nonexistent or too small to mean much.

Community collaborations by their nature are usually complex and often large in size. Over the life of a local effort, any one funder's dollar contribution is likely to be relatively small. Partners must take care to identify the most effective role for the funder to play. In the end, the funder–community collaboration partnership must be one that honors the values of community residents intended to be affected by the local effort.

"People are empowered," John H. Stanfield II said in a 1999 *American Journal of Evaluation* article,

> when they have the power to contribute to the operations and transformation of the institutions that employ them, the institutions in which they otherwise participate, and the communities in which they live, work, and play. They are not empowered when they are simply invited to participate or work or play in an institution in which they lack influential access to key decision-making roles and circles. (p. 427)

This is not to say, however, any idea that is local is worthy of funder support. An idea's origin cannot be its validation. Local leaders who regularly petition funders may be as out of step with neighborhood residents as the stereotypical foundation. Further, foundations with long experience in supporting community collaborations can draw on a reliable history of local practice as a guide. Indeed, one of the biggest mistakes a funder makes is ignoring its own experiences. The field is awash with so-called lessons learned, but, to paraphrase evaluator Michael Quinn Patton, there is little evidence to substantiate the allegation that we have learned something.

At the foundation where I work, our recent experience in supporting planning and implementation projects with community collaborations yields several lessons that will guide us going forward. Here are five.

1.   *There is no distinct planning phase; planning has no clear start and stop date.* Most of all, planning does not occur in place of action. Borrowing Donald Campbell's idea that social experimentation requires an "active society," community collaborations must create and use their own feedback and monitoring systems to help stakeholders undertake activities designed to yield short- and long-term results (Campbell, 1998). As Campbell said: "Faced with a choice between innovating a new program or commissioning a thorough study of the problem as a prelude to action, the bias would be toward innovating" (p. 13). A common mistake among funders and nonprofits is the attempt to plan under one set of values and implement under another.

At Knight Foundation, we often see influential community groups whose appetite for local reconnaissance and research gets in the way of implementation. This seemingly endless planning can tire out local practitioners who prefer action. Our recent economic development grant making in Grand Forks, North Dakota, provides an example of how we have handled this. We used a fast-response approach in our local reconnaissance, sending a team of staff and economic development experts to Grand Forks, in May 2001, to interview more than three dozen elites over 2 days. The culmination of the second day was a staff presentation back to the group. Within 2 months, we followed up by hosting local meetings of working groups. By fall 2001, we made our first set of economic development grants in the community. The local planning continues, but it is integrated into the community's action, and local leaders have taken ownership.

2. *Funders must invest time and resources to communicate effectively with their community-based partners.* Messages that foundation staff believe to be simple and direct may come across as ambiguous and inconsistent. Local leaders may perceive that different foundation staff send different signals. Indeed, staff may be doing just that. It takes time and, most of all, trust, for funders and community collaborations to speak candidly about issues related to grant dollars, evaluation, and the need for midterm corrections. The need for clear and effective communication between funder and community collaboration does not end with the grant award.

3. *Funders can provide resources other than dollars.* Old-fashioned networking (called "convening" these days) can help local leaders learn from their peers in other communities and can open the door to valuable expertise and even additional grant dollars. To realize these benefits, funders need to be nimble enough to respond to shifting moods and circumstances. Again, relationships are the key. Funders cannot pop in once a year and offer to convene partners in a local collaboration. At best, nonprofits will view this as an annoyance. Funders must immerse themselves in the community, so that staff can move quickly when opportunities arise. This is about more than meeting for the sake of meeting. Through his work with several communities, for example, Richard Harwood has figured out ways to make networking and convening systematic. A publication from the Harwood Institute, *Community Rhythms: Five Stages of Community Life* (1999), describes how community leaders can use a reflective process to determine their current stage of growth. Harwood's design helps communities place themselves on a continuum of growth that ranges from stagnation (what Harwood calls "The Waiting Place") to maintenance, or what he calls "Sustain/Renew." "Only if you know and understand the stage at which our community rests," Harwood writes, "will you be better able to figure out what kinds of approaches, strategies and timing best fit for your seeking to move your community forward" (p. 9).

4. *Funders and community collaborations must agree at the outset on the outcomes for which the joint effort will be held accountable.* Turning again to Campbell (1998), stakeholders must remember that determining "hard-headed, multidimensional evaluations of outcomes" (p. 11) is the only way to build upon successes and improve upon failures. Whether a funder supports a narrow slice of the collaboration's overall work or provides general operating support with no strings attached, the anticipated outcomes must be explicit from the start. The temptation to gray the lines, in order to make the grant, which often occurs when there are time pressures, increases the likelihood of frustration later in the process, when one or both sets of stakeholders clarifies its own expectations and realizes the partnership is a bad fit.

We are living through a great example of this right now at Knight Foundation. In June 2001, we made a collection of large community development grants in Miami, which, at the time, appeared pretty well organized. Only after the grants were made, when the nitty-gritty work of the partnership began, did we become aware of our lack of detailed focus on benchmarks and outcomes. It is difficult to make up that lost ground. The truism here is that it is better to figure these things out before a grant is made, rather than after. Funders need to be clear and candid about expectations they bring to the partnership. Likewise, discussing the risks they face is critical for funders and community collaborations, and potential risks should be balanced against the potential returns. The worst case, as Lisbeth Schorr (1999) points out, is to proceed without reconciling these expectations:

> An unrelenting focus on real results exposes the sham of asking human-service providers, educators, and community organizers to accomplish massive tasks with wholly inadequate resources and tools. It forces the question of whether to expect less from limited investments—or to invest more to operate at the level of intensity that is necessary to achieve promised results. (p. 42)

5. *Instead of focusing only on the search for evidence of causation* (what evaluator Michael Quinn Patton [1986] calls the elusiveness of "definitive, pound-your-fist-on-the-table conclusions" [p. 217]), *funders working with community collaborations on social change strategies should first examine the long list of assumptions that drive their thinking.* Funders need to invest the time and energy needed to build strong theory for their investments. "When the evaluator seeks to elicit foundations of program theory from those engaged in the initiatives," as Carol Weiss says, "they

may begin to see some of the leaps of faith that are embedded in it" (Weiss, 1995, p. 72).

At Knight Foundation, for instance, we have been working with child care providers in an urban setting, to identify strategies that would improve staff retention. High turnover among child care professionals helps deprive children of a stable environment and consistent relationships with adults. The obvious incentive is money. But our discussions of the underlying assumptions have convinced us that the situation is more complicated. Is the relatively small amount of money we could provide to supplement staff salaries going to convince child care professionals to remain in their current positions? Perhaps they leave for other reasons, such as a poor benefits package, little room for professional advancement, or stress associated with the job. We have not sorted out the answers, but the deliberations are strengthening our work.

REFERENCES

Campbell, D. T. (1998). The experimenting society. In W. N. Dunn (Ed.), *The experimenting society: Essays in honor of Donald T. Campbell* (pp. 9–45). New Brunswick, NJ: Transaction Publishers, 1998.

Harwood Group (1999). *Community rhythms: Five stages of community life.* A report prepared for The Mott Foundation. Bethesda, MD: Author.

Patton, M. Q. (1986). *Utilization-focused evaluation.* Beverly Hills, CA: Sage.

Schorr, L. (1999). Changing the rules: The key to expanding what works, *Chronicle of Philanthropy, 11*(22), 42–43.

Stanfield, J. H., II (1999). Slipping through the front door: Relevant social scientific evaluation in the people of color. *Century American Journal of Evaluation, 20*(3), 415–431.

Weiss, C. H. (1995). Nothing as practical as good theory: Exploring theory-based evaluation for Comprehensive Community Initiatives for Children and Families. In J. P. Connell, A. C. Kubisch, L. Schon, & C. H. Weiss (Eds.), *New approaches to evaluating community initiatives: Concepts, methods, and contexts* (pp. 65–92). Washington, DC: The Aspen Institute.

Index